D1292251

HYSTERIA

HYSTERIA

The Biography

———∞∞∞———

Andrew Scull

OXFORD
UNIVERSITY PRESS

OXFORD

UNIVERSITY PRESS

Great Clarendon Street, Oxford OX2 6DP

Oxford University Press is a department of the University of Oxford.
It furthers the University's objective of excellence in research, scholarship,
and education by publishing worldwide in

Oxford New York

Auckland Cape Town Dar es Salaam Hong Kong Karachi
Kuala Lumpur Madrid Melbourne Mexico City Nairobi
New Delhi Shanghai Taipei Toronto

With offices in

Argentina Austria Brazil Chile Czech Republic France Greece
Guatemala Hungary Italy Japan Poland Portugal Singapore
South Korea Switzerland Thailand Turkey Ukraine Vietnam

Oxford is a registered trade mark of Oxford University Press
in the UK and in certain other countries

Published in the United States
by Oxford University Press Inc., New York

British Library Cataloguing in Publication Data

Data available

Library of Congress Cataloging-in-Publication Data

Scull, Andrew T.
Hysteria : the biography / Andrew Scull.
p.; cm.
Includes bibliographical references and index.
ISBN 978-0-19-956096-7 (hardback : alk. paper) 1. Hysteria—History. I. Title.
[DNLM: 1. Hysteria—history. 2. History, Modern 1601-. WM 11.1 S437h 2009]
RC532.S38 2009
616.85'24—dc22   2009026410

Typeset by SPI Publisher Services, Pondicherry, India
Printed in Great Britain
on acid-free paper by
Clays Ltd, St Ives plc

ISBN 978–0–19–956096–7

1 3 5 7 9 10 8 6 4 2

CONTENTS

LIST OF ILLUSTRATIONS

PROLOGUE:

Suffocation of the Mother

London, Friday, April 30, 1602. The last year of Elizabeth I's reign. A 14-year-old girl, Mary Glover, the daughter of a well-to-do shopkeeper, left her house on Thames Street to run an errand for her mother. She soon arrived at her destination, the house of Elizabeth Jackson, a neighbor with whom she had quarreled in the past, where she sought to deliver her message. Seizing the opportunity, however, the old woman drew the teenager indoors, "locked the dore upon her," and rained down imprecations and threats on the young girl's head, cursing her for damaging her reputation in the community and for meddling with her own daughter's apparel, and "wishing an evil death to light upon her." For upwards of an hour, the old crone ranted and raved at Mary, till finally she relented and let her go, with the parting injunction that "My daughter shall have clothes when thou art dead and rotten."[1]

Understandably, the encounter left young Mary pale and shaken. Savoring her triumph, Elizabeth Jackson crowed to a servant in the house next door, Elizabeth Burges, that she had "ratled up" the young creature, and added: "I hope an evill death will come unto her."[2] On the following Monday, apparently

1

not content with her first round of curses, Jackson showed up at the Glovers' shop, ostensibly to see Mary's mother. Glaring and snarling at the girl as she sat drinking a posset, she spoke harshly to her, then abruptly turned on her heel and left.

Immediately seized by a choking sensation, Mary found she could no longer swallow her posset. Her throat seemed to swell and close, though not enough to inhibit her breathing. She went to a family friend for help, only to find herself "speechles and blynde."[3] Brought back to her father, she continued to have fits three and four times a day. By Wednesday, "her fittes were so fearfull, that all that were about her, supposed that she would dye." Her parents asked that the church bells "be touled for her," and hearing the sound, Elizabeth Jackson rushed next door rejoicing. "I thank my God," she announced, "he hath heard my prayer, and stopped the mouth and tyed the tongue of one of myne enemies…The vengeance of God on her and on all the generation of them."[4]

God's vengeance apparently did not stretch so far as to cause Mary's demise, but over the following weeks, the fits continued, and eventually got worse. Eating proved difficult. To keep her alive, nutrients were periodically thrust down Mary's throat. (She had developed a preternatural capacity to have fingers or instruments thrust far down her gullet without gagging.) Next, she developed a paralysis of a hand, then an arm, and then of her whole left side. Her belly swelled. Further periods of blindness and inability to speak were accompanied by more swelling of the throat. The fits seemed worse every other day, but always came on when she tried to eat.

On two occasions she encountered Mistress Jackson, first in the shop, and then at church, after which her symptoms took a still more dramatic turn:

she was turned rounde as a whoop [hoop], with her head backward to her hippes; and in that position rolled and tumbled, with such violence, and swiftness, as that their paynes in keeping her from receaving hurt against the bedsted, and postes, caused two or three women to sweat; she being all over colde and stiffe as a frozen thing. After she had ben thus tossed and tumbled in this circled roundnes backward, her body was suddenly turned round the contrary way, that is, her head forward betweene her leggs, and then also rowled and tumbled as before.[5]

The weeks that followed were beset with other writhings and contortions of the body; dancings and prancings; movements in slow motion into postures that seemed impossible to sustain; strange patterns of breathing and alterations of countenance; "many strange anticke formes" of the mouth, "distortions, gapings and blastings," accompanied by odd vocalizations; while, at other times, she mimed shooting a bow and arrow or plucking at the strings of a harp, yet seemed "dumbe, blynde, and senseless."[6] In the midst of her fits, she at times shouted out her gratitude to God, and called upon Him to deliver her from her afflictions. As word spread of these dramatic posturings, crowds of pious Puritans, augmented by the skeptical and the curious, gathered to view the spectacle.

Finally, after some weeks, Glover was brought to the Sheriff's house to meet face-to-face with the woman whose imprecations had coincided with the origins of her torments. It was one of several such meetings, all accompanied by still more spectacular and frightening outbursts, physical and verbal, that lasted for hours: paralyses, trances, tics, spasms, and contortions that resembled a creature possessed; roaring cries and grimaces; exhibitions of torment that served to "make her a like terror to all beholders" (p. 14); invocations of the Almighty;

a shrinking from contact with Elizabeth Jackson; and, at the height of the drama,

> the mouth being fast shut, and her lipps close, there cam a voice through her nostrills, that sounded very like (especially at som time) Hange her, or Honge her. The repetition whereof, never ceased, so long as that Elizabeth Jackson was to be found within the compas of that roofe; and she no sooner departed the house, but the voice ceased presently.[7]

What to make of it all? Sensing that Mary's reactions might all be a carefully contrived act, those around her tried a number of experiments to expose the counterfeit. Both Glover and Jackson were ordered to appear before Mr Crooke, the Recorder of London, at his rooms in the Inner Temple. Mary Glover was brought in first. Crooke then resorted to a subterfuge:

> he choose out a woman both aged, homely, grosse bodyed, and of lowe stature, very comparable to Elizabeth Jackson. Her did he cause to put on Elizabeth Jacksons hatt, and a muffler on her face, and then brought her up to the chamber where Mary Glover was, caused Mary to walke by her, two or three returnes, and to touch the woman once....[8]

Nothing. Then, the first woman having left the room, Elizabeth Jackson appeared, disguised in the clothes of another. At once, the fits returned, along with the voice through the nostrils demanding that Jackson be hanged. Seeing Glover apparently senseless, the Recorder called for a candle, and brought the flame up to her cheek, and then near to her eyes, as though to burn and blind her. Glover's wide-eyed stare was unblinking. He called for some pieces of paper, crumpled them up, and lit them, thrusting the burning objects one after another into the palm of her right hand. No reaction was forthcoming (though, when Glover recovered from her fit, her hand was visibly burned "in five severall places"). "When he saw this setled insensibilitie, he proved the fyre upon [Jackson's] hand, who cryed upon him not to burne her...Then Mr Recorder caused Elizabeth Jackson to kneele downe, and say the Lords prayer: therein (as she ever used to doe) she skipped *Deliver us from evill...,*" upon which her teenage accuser convulsed, and, in a strange nasal voice, again called out "hang her, hang her."[9]

How was one to make sense of these dramatic events? For large numbers of Glover and Jackson's contemporaries, occupying a world where God and the Devil were omnipresent, where the supernatural and natural worlds overlapped and constantly collided, the meanings to attach to this narrative were obvious. Mary Glover's actions and reactions were those of a person bewitched or diabolically possessed. And the source of her possession was none other than Elizabeth Jackson, who stood revealed as the witch who had cast a spell on her, the agent of the Devil himself.

Such was the judgment of *hoi polloi,* soon ratified in legal proceedings. Arraigned before the Chief Justice of the Court of Common Pleas, Sir Edmund Anderson, and a number of other judges, the illiterate old woman stood accused of being a witch. Anderson was notorious as a witch-finding judge, heightening the old woman's peril. Yet at the trial not all were convinced of her guilt, and Jackson was not without her defenders. A number of the spectators clearly sided with her and viewed her adolescent accuser as a counterfeit and a fraud. Anderson would have none of it. Elizabeth Jackson was guilty as charged, and sentenced to a year's imprisonment, and to stand several times in the pillory.

I

∞∞∞∞

MYSTERIA

E lizabeth Jackson's conviction for witchcraft was not the end of the story. As we shall soon see, a radically different interpretation of Mary Glover's afflictions had been proffered at her trial. The judge rejected that testimony, as did the jury. But it was an alternative account that had a long pedigree, and its proponent was a respectable man with powerful political allies. Mary was not bewitched, but hysterical, or so it was alleged. Where had that term come from? What is that disorder, whose biography is our subject?

Hysteria is a pathological condition with a fascinating and tortuous medical and cultural history. If the malady seems to change its shape and its form over the centuries, who can be surprised? For here is a disorder that even those who insist on its reality concede is a chameleon-like disease that can mimic the symptoms of any other, and one that somehow seems to mold itself to the culture in which it appears.

The nineteenth-century American neurologist and novelist Silas Weir Mitchell invented what was once the most widely used treatment for this affliction, his famous rest cure, and grew

rich on the proceeds from the hundreds of hysterics who annu-
ally crowded into his Philadelphia consulting rooms. Yet, like
most of his medical colleagues, he pronounced himself baffled
by much of what he saw: the trances, the fits, the paralyses, the
choking, the tearing of hair, the remarkable emotional instability, all with no obvious organic substrate. Hysteria was "the
nosological limbo of all un-named female maladies," a condition that so challenged his powers of understanding and his
therapeutic skills that he often referred to it in tones of exas-
peration as "mysteria."[1] Like the doctors who once despaired
of its mysteries, perhaps the historian who ventures to write
the biography of so elusive a subject will learn to rue the day
he or she ventured upon such a Sisyphean task. Hence surely
Edward Shorter's lament: "Writing a history of something so
amorphous, whose meaning and content keep changing, is like
trying to write a history of dirt."[2] But it is also possible to revel in
hysteria's ambiguities and contradictions, as I prefer to do.

Was hysteria "real" or fictitious, somatic or psychopathologic-
al? Might it constitute an unspoken idiom of protest, a symbolic
voice for the silenced sex, who were forbidden to verbalize their
discontents, and so created a language of the body? Perhaps it
was simply an elaborate ruse, a complex kind of malingering
and manipulation that rendered its baffling, infuriating patients
worthy of blame and punishment? Or, in the alternative, was
it no more than a diagnostic waste bin, a heterogeneous congeries of complaints cobbled together linguistically, mostly a
testimony to medical myth-making, incomprehension, and
ignorance? At various times, and sometimes simultaneously, all
of these claims have had their advocates. It is small wonder that
the prominent mid-twentieth-century British psychiatrist Eliot
Slater spoke contemptuously of the diagnosis as "a disguise for

ignorance and a fertile source of clinical error ... not only a delusion but also a snare."[3]

How, in the face of such contradictions and uncertainties, are we to proceed? How can we define the very subject of our inquiry? It does no good to declare that one's subject is "behavior that produces the *appearance* of disease." Not only does that avoid one of the questions at issue, but it does so in a way that requires us to second-guess doctors and patients throughout most of human history. Certainly, by the twentieth century, most doctors had convinced themselves that hysteria was a psychological disorder, "an affliction of the mind that was expressed through a disturbance of the body."[4] But, for centuries before, physicians had insisted that hysteria was a "real" somatic disorder, and those suffering from hysterical afflictions have continued so to insist, for the most part, right up to the present. And sometimes the patients are proved right: in the heyday of psychoanalysis, all sorts of complaints that had been diagnosed as hysterical were subsequently proved to have a physiological cause, a category mistake that could have profound, even fatal, consequences for the individuals concerned.[5]

Moreover, the perils of retrospective diagnoses of what was "really" wrong with patients in the past are clear. Second-guessing that is little more than speculation is never very helpful. So, by and large, mine is a biography of what contemporaries saw and interpreted as hysteria. I accept that, as with other diagnoses from the past, our still fallible contemporary versions of medical science might now assign them to very different categories of disease. Even choosing this option, though, does not provide a neat solution to the dilemma of what to include in the hysterical universe.

In a variety of historical settings, the decision about whether to apply the hysterical label was essentially a contested one, never finally resolved. In others, an alternative medical label was proffered, though whether the distinctions in question were real and substantial was acknowledged to be doubtful, even at the time. Thus, in the seventeenth and eighteenth centuries, there was much anguishing about the distinctions between hysteria, hypochondria, the spleen, and the vapors, though for many informed physicians this was seen as so much hair-splitting, rather than corresponding to a clearly separable set of disorders. In the late nineteenth century, the construction of neurasthenia, or weakness of the nerves, was similarly controversial. Some alleged that it was a subterfuge to create a label more acceptable to men who shrank from being called hysterical (though, confusingly, there were a multitude of female neurasthenics). Others simply adopted the term as a convenient fiction, while cheerfully acknowledging that there was no clear dividing line between hysteria and neurasthenia. In the First World War, "shell shock" was originally thought to be a neurological disorder. Only later did most (but by no means all) informed medical opinion on both sides of the conflict come around to the view that it was an epidemic of male hysteria. And, in our own time, disputes rage about whether such entities as "chronic fatigue syndrome," Gulf War syndrome, and myalgic encephalomyelitis are merely a modern manifestation of hysteria, or "genuine" illnesses. Such ambiguities and roiling disputes are part and parcel of the strange biography of hysteria, and, rather than ignore them, I have chosen to make them a central part of the narrative that follows.

The biography of such a disease, if disease it be, obviously cannot be reduced to a simple story. Not that others haven't tried.

For the Freudians, hysteria is the quintessential psychodynamic disorder, and its history a tale of fallacious medical materialism alternating with superstitious attributions of spirit possession and demonology, occasionally interrupted by brave pioneers who reject both forms of prejudice and perceive its true, psychological origins. Enlightenment finally triumphs with the advent of Sigmund Freud. For the famous critic of contemporary psychiatry Thomas Szasz, the very recognition of hysteria's non-somatic origins is proof that it does not deserve the status of a disease, but is instead the *locus classicus* of the medical manufacture of madness, with doctor and patient down through history playing an elaborate, bad-faith game. Mental illness, Szasz proclaims, is a myth, and hysteria perhaps the most telling illustration of the mythological character of psychiatry's proclamations. I shall advance no such simplicities here.

Many—indeed most—of the diseases we currently recognize have appeared since the beginning of the nineteenth century. That should occasion no surprise. For those committed to the notion of medicine as a developing science, it seems obvious that, as that science advances, its conceptions of etiology and pathology evolve, new discoveries force the reassessment of traditional categories, and an ever more complex account and classification of diseases result.

All save the most doctrinaire proponents of the idea that disease is socially constructed will concede that there is much to be said for this account. As our understanding of our bodies has grown, such broad categories as cardiac or pulmonary disease, or diseases of the nervous system, have inevitably been elaborated into more and more complex arrays of disorders, many of them named after those who "discovered" them (or occasionally, as with Amyotrophic Lateral Sclerosis, or Lou Gehrig's disease, named after those who were unfortunate enough to suffer from them). One may adopt a more sociologically sophisticated perspective on these developments, noting that disease categories may be politicized (as with the construction and deconstruction of homosexuality as a disease), and that decisions to construct diseases in particular ways are often debatable and negotiated. Rather than timeless entities that "cut nature at the joints," disease entities are complex cultural productions. They depend upon layers of interpretation being placed upon whatever underlying physiological and psychological disturbances give rise to them. As such, they (and their boundaries) are inevitably subject to contestation and renegotiation, and not just because of the accumulation of new "knowledge." The fundamental point remains: the realm of disease is unstable, with etiologies and nosologies always exhibiting some degree of flux, and doctors are generally no more able than their patients to shake themselves free of the assumptions and prejudices of their era.

And there is another reason why most diseases date from the past two centuries: till then, Western medicine shied away from the notion of disease specificity. Indeed, the promotion of such notions was often seen as one of the characteristics of quacks and charlatans. For millennia, disease was viewed in a holistic way, as the product of systematic disturbances in the balance of forces that characterized each of us. Diagnosis and treatment were a matter of working out where the balance of humors had gone astray, and deciding how to bring them back into equilibrium.

Doctors from the early nineteenth century onward were eager to tie their nosologies and diagnoses to observations at the bedside or, still more persuasively, findings in the laboratory.

In earlier centuries, however, appeals to the canonical texts of Hippocrates and Galen were standard ways of legitimizing diseases and their treatments. In linking particular diseases to these authorities, medical men in early modern Europe (and the patients who embraced their nostrums) were connecting their ideas and practices to a tenacious, broadly shared, and authoritative universe of meanings, beliefs, and behaviors. And certain features of their medical cosmology made the promulgation of the disease of hysteria plausible to themselves and those they treated. Their notions of health and disease set up no firm division between body and environment, the local and the systemic, soma and psyche, each element in these dyads being capable of influencing the other. The part and the whole were inseparable and inextricably tied together, with disequilibrium in any corner or cranny threatening the equilibrium (and thus the health) of anybody or any body.

Here was a set of culturally shared understandings of the sources of disease and of its therapeutics that persisted with very little change for centuries. The body was held to be a system in constant dynamic interaction with its environment, so tightly interconnected that local lesions produced systemic effects. Seasonal changes as well as developmental crises over the course of a lifetime constantly threatened the equilibrium of the system, and thus the health of the patient. Bodies assimilated and excreted, and were affected by diet, exercise, and regimen, as well as pre-existing constitutional endowment, all of which might change the balance of the humors and thus the health, physical and mental, of the patient. Upset bodies produced upset minds, and vice versa. It was the job of the physician to recognize why the equilibrium that was good health had been thrown out of kilter, and then to mobilize the tools at his disposal to affect a readjustment of the patient's internal state. Ritually reaffirmed through the therapeutic encounter, "the system provided a rationalistic framework in which the physician could at once reassure the patient and legitimate his own ministrations."[6]

Women were different. Of that there could be no doubt. And the differences were consequential for their health. Hence the disposition of physicians in the ancient world to place women's reproductive systems at the heart of accounting for their susceptibility to all sorts of disease and debility. In women, so one Hippocratic text read, "the womb is the origin of all diseases." It was not just that the female of the species was differently constituted from the male; she was also fundamentally inferior: moister, looser textured, softer, with spongier flesh. Her body was more readily deranged—for example, by puberty, pregnancy, or parturition, by menopause, or by suppressed menstruation, all of which could impose profound shocks on her internal equilibrium (for her wetter constitution produced an excess of blood, which regularly needed to be drained from her system); or by the womb wandering about internally in search of moisture (or, later, sending forth vapors that rose through the body), disturbances that were held to be the source of a great variety of organic complaints. It was from these notions, reworked by Galen and other Roman commentators, and for the most part re-entering the West from Arabic medicine in the Renaissance, that the classical accounts of hysteria were constructed.

Plato's *Timaeus*, in George Rousseau's vivid précis, had viewed "the womb as an animal: voracious, predatory, appetitive, unstable, forever reducing the female into a frail and unstable creature."[7] Many medical writers of the Classical Age were not inclined to disagree. Certainly, as Helen King has done much to establish, the presence of a full-blown clinical description of hysteria in the Hippocratic texts is a modern fable, but the notions of a wandering womb, and of women's gynecology as the source of a multitude of mental and physical ills, can certainly be found there. And they were amplified and debated in the Roman era.

Celsus and Aretaeus, closely associated with the Hippocratic tradition, both adopted the notion of the womb wandering about the abdomen, stirring up all manner of troubles. If it migrated upward, for example, it compressed other bodily organs, producing a sense of choking, even a loss of speech. "Sometimes," Celsus claimed, "this affection deprives the patient of all sensibility, in the same manner as if she had fallen in epilepsia. Yet with this difference, that neither the eyes are turned, nor does foam flow from the mouth, nor are there any convulsions: there is only a profound sleep."[8] Both Soranus and Galen, by contrast, disputed the notion that the womb could wander, though they accepted that it was the organ from which hysterical symptoms derived. These manifestations of the disease could take a multitude of forms: extreme emotionality; but also a variety of physical disturbances, ranging from simple dizziness, through paralyses, and respiratory distress. Then there was the commonly reported sensation of a ball in the throat, constricting breathing and creating a sense of suffocation, the so-called *globus hystericus*.

There was thus a venerable tradition within Western medicine that linked hysteria to gender—and perhaps even to sexuality, for Galen held that sexual deprivation could cause the disorder, and advocated intercourse for the married, and marriage for the single, as a frequently valuable therapeutic tactic.

It was a tradition that firmly located an array of strange bodily symptoms that others might be tempted to attribute to the supernatural—to bewitchment, or to possession by devils—to the material universe, and to disorders of the female body. And it was a tradition that was invoked for the first time in an English courtroom at the dawn of the Jacobean age.

The trial of Elizabeth Jackson had led, as we saw in the Prologue, to her conviction for bewitching young Mary Glover, a conviction that for many contemporaries was amply warranted by the facts. But she had had a defender who was not from her neighborhood, nor one of the audience who considered young Mary a counterfeit and a fraud, nor one of her class or background at all. Instead, one of England's medical elite had taken the witness stand, and he had tried to invoke what authority his profession possessed to rebut claims of witchcraft and to provide what he claimed was an explanation sanctioned by Galen and Hippocrates.

Curiously, as it may seem at first, Edward Jorden, an influential member of London's College of Physicians, had chosen to appear on poor widow Jackson's behalf. The burden of Jorden's testimony, and of a subsequent pamphlet he published on the case, was that Mary Glover suffered from "hysterica passio" or "suffocation of the mother."[9] Hers was an instance not of demonic possession, but of a bodily illness. It belonged, in other words, to the world of the natural, not the supernatural. Accordingly, Elizabeth Jackson was wholly innocent of the charge of witchcraft.

In support of his claims, Jorden was quick to point to women's greater susceptibility to disease, and to their particular susceptibility to the "suffocation of the mother," because of the womb's close connections with "the braine, heart, and liver…and the easie passage which it hath into them by the Vaines, Arteries,

A BRIEFE DIS-COVRSE OF A DIS-EASE CALLED THE

Suffocation of the *Mother*.

Written vppon occasion which hath beene of late taken thereby, to suspect possession of an euill spirit, or some such like supernaturall power.

Wherin is declared that diuers strange actions and passions of the body of man, which in *the common opinion, are imputed to the Diuell, haue their true naturall causes, and do accompanie this disease.*

By EDVVARD IORDEN

Doctor in Physicke.

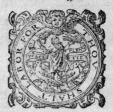

LONDON.

Printed by Iohn Windet, dwelling at the Signe of the Crosse Keyes at Powles Wharfe. 1 6 0 3.

1. *The Suffocation of the Mother.* Title page of Edward Jorden's pamphlet. (*Wellcome Library, London*)

and Nerves."[10] Here was a disease whose symptoms were "monstrous and terrible to beholde, and of such a varietie as they can hardly be comprehended within any method or boundes"— and liable to deceive the credulous and the unlearned, who all-too-readily ascribe them "either to diabolicall possession, to witchcraft, or to the immediate finger of the Almightie."[11] One particularly common affliction was a sense of "suffocation in the throate."[12] Hence the disease's common vernacular name.

But, in arguing for the protean quality of hysterical complaints, Jorden was opening himself up to ridicule and rebuttal. In the course of his testimony he was asked whether he could cure Glover, and he confessed he could not. Would he treat her? No, he would not. Was Glover counterfeiting and a fraud? No, she was not. (It would have been difficult for Jorden to assent to this last query, for not long before, in front of the judges, Mary had once more been accused of faking her symptoms, and had had her hand severely burned, an ordeal she bore without blinking or evident sign of distress.)

Disdainfully, Sir Edmund Anderson dismissed Jorden's testimony: "Then in my conscience, it is not naturall; for if you tell me neither a Naturall cause of it, nor a naturall remedy, I will tell you, that it is not naturall ... I care not for your Judgement."[13] Instructing the jury, he pointed out that widow Jackson had stumbled once more over the words of the Lord's Prayer and the Creed, and bore on her body the witch's mark. "Phisitions [Physicians]," however "learned and wise," had confessed their ignorance of both cause and cure: "geve me a naturall reason, and a naturall remedy, or a rush for your phisicke."[14]

The jury, who doubtless shared Anderson's view of the world, had no hesitation in convicting, and the judge had no hesitation in sentencing Jackson to prison and the pillory. But it was a sentence Jackson would never serve, for her influential supporters quickly secured her release. In a way, one might say that she was doubly fortunate, for she had been convicted under the relatively lenient terms of the Witchcraft Act of 1563. Two years after her trial, the law was revised, and even witchcraft that did not result in the victim's death became a capital offense.

Spurned in the courtroom, Edward Jorden was not yet done with the case. Within months, he had produced and published a lengthy pamphlet spelling out for his readers the etiology and symptoms of "a disease called the Suffocation of the Mother," afflictions that "in the common opinion, are imputed to the Devill."[15] Where before he had vacillated on the question of whether Mary Glover had been a fraud, he now emphatically denied it. It was an affliction of her uterus and subsequently of her brain that had brought on her symptoms, and it was thus to medicine, not the interventions of divines, that one should look for a cure.

> For if it be true that one man cannot be perfect in every arte and profession…Why should we not prefer the judgements of Phisitions in a question concerning the actions and passions of mans [sic] body (the proper subject of that profession) before our owne conceites; as we do the opinions of Divines, Lawyers, Artificers, &c. in their proper Elements.[16]

Foul and fragrant smells, tight lacing, and a sparing diet could and should be employed to calm and remove the fits.

It was an opinion largely ignored or rejected in its day. Mary Glover had continued to have fits, even after Jackson's conviction, till her parents, pious and prominent Puritans, summoned divines and the devout to her bedside to pray and to fast, and so to cast out "her devills." A day of struggle supervened. As the assembled believers prayed over the young girl, her body acted out her inner turmoil. She was wracked by convulsions and contortions, which grew in intensity till the climatic moment arrived, and the devil seemed to leave her, as she cried out that God had come and that the Lord had delivered her. For her Puritan audience, the proof of her possession could not have been clearer, for those were the very words her grandfather had uttered as he burned to death at the stake, the victim of the "Papists" unleashed during the Catholic reign of terror that accompanied Queen Mary's brief tenure on the English throne. Their religion, their God, had been vindicated by Mary Glover's case, and Satan cast out of her body.

As the historian Michael MacDonald has shown, it was this very ritual of dispossession that had prompted the appearance of Edward Jorden's pamphlet. As Jorden himself confessed in its opening lines, "I have not undertaken this businesse of mine own accord."[17] Instead, he had been commissioned to write it by the Bishop of London, Richard Bancroft. To modern eyes, the text looks like an effort to forward the claims of a secular naturalism ranged against the traditional claims of religion. In reality, however, MacDonald argues that it was first and foremost itself a piece of religious propaganda, forming part of the two-front war orthodox Anglicans were engaged in: on the one hand, against the Jesuits and other agents of idolatrous Popery; and, on the other, against the claims of a clamorous band of Puritans bent on recruiting the English state to their cause. The stakes were all the higher, because the death of Queen Elizabeth had brought to the throne James, the King of Scotland, a man who had previously demonstrated his own enthusiasm for *Daemonologie* in his 1597 pamphlet with that title.

Both Catholics and Puritans used what they saw as miracles to advance the legitimacy and authority of their faith: Jesuits could rely upon an elaborate ritual of exorcism to eliminate super-natural afflictions, and had performed some spectacular and well-publicized rites, the driving-out of demons proving potent propaganda for their cause. Their Puritan opponents, dismissing the Papist ceremonies as superstitious nonsense bereft of biblical authority, nonetheless invoked a passage in the Gospel of Mark, where Jesus supposedly attributed His cure of a youth afflicted with a "deaf and dumb spirit" to the power of prayer and fasting, to justify developing their own weapon against Satan's wiles. Fearful of both religious extremes, the English state had tried straightforward repression of both groups, banning books, and imprisoning practitioners. Jorden's text represented a different tack in the same struggle, an intellectual counter-blast designed to discredit both forms of exorcism, and thereby to weaken the appeal of those practicing them.

Bancroft, and his aged superior, John Whitgift, whom he would succeed as Archbishop of Canterbury, were rightly notorious for their rigid intolerance of Puritans. Fortunately for them, they seem to have succeeded in persuading King James to share their hatred for "insolent Puritanes" as well as "superstitious Priests," the twinned enemies of true religion who were the targets of his wrath in his 1604 *Counterblast to Tobacco*. Bancroft introduced Jorden to the King, and not long after, and perhaps not coincidentally, James abandoned his earlier enthusiasm for witch-hunting, preferring instead to make sport of exposing frauds and imposters pretending to be possessed.

In that sense, Jorden's arguments won the day, at least at the level of high politics, and one might even argue that they indirectly played a role in the diminution and eventual disappearance of the legal persecution of "witches." Elsewhere, however, it was a different story. Repressed they might be, but Puritans and their sympathizers continued throughout the seventeenth century to circulate the story of little Mary Glover, her possession and dispossession. It was a triumph for, and a testimony to, the truth of their religious convictions. And, among his fellow physicians, Jorden's pamphlet was little noticed, and soon forgotten. Even when he wrote it, many of his colleagues in the College of Physicians had signaled their belief that Mary Glover was indeed bewitched. *A Briefe Discourse of a Disease Called the Suffocation of the Mother* had but a short half-life and then disappeared from view, never reprinted, seldom cited, left to the gnawing criticism of the mice. With it went any serious interest in the disease it claimed to identify, and that interest would not revive for several decades.

And yet, Mary Glover's case displays some remarkable features, phenomena that we shall encounter again and again as we trace the curious career of the now-vanished disease known as hysteria. Take her symptoms, for example. Loss of speech and sight, and an inability to swallow; paralyses of hands, arms, legs; mysterious swellings of the abdomen or throat; a sense of suffocation; odd breathing patterns; loss of sensation and of reflex action—all these are classic recurrent features of something, a putative syndrome that in later centuries came to be seen as the manifestation of hysteria. Then there are the assumptions of odd postures and facial expressions, the writhings and contortions, and the strange vocal tics. These, too, we shall encounter in some very different settings. As for the preternatural ability to transform one's body into a circle and roll around the room like a human wheel, performances of this sort, labeled the *arc-en-cercle*, would become one of the features of the hysterical circus to which the eminent neurologist Jean-Martin Charcot would serve as ring-master in late-nineteenth-century Paris.

Above all, of course, there is the dramatic character of all these symptoms, the striking impression they made on any and all who had occasion to witness them, arousing the persistent suspicion that what was being watched was in reality an act.

That many medical men should profess themselves baffled by these strange manifestations, and that some would deny that what they were observing was a natural disease, is again a feature we shall observe repeating itself. Many suspected that Mary Glover was faking her symptoms. Even Edward Jorden at times seems to have joined the ranks of the skeptics. Many of Mary's symptoms aroused suspicion, and seemed conveniently calculated to take revenge on the old woman who had abused and frightened her. If Elizabeth Jackson wanted her dead, she would respond in kind: "Hang her, hang her." Perhaps it was all an elaborate act, a malingering, a calculated use of bodily symptoms to gain social advantage. These, too, would be familiar features of the disorder, as would the failure of threats and even the infliction of severe pain to have a discernible effect on the sufferer.

And yet, if it was all an act, how was Mary Glover able to endure the burning of her flesh, or the approach of a flame that seemed destined to blind her? The mass psychiatric casualties of a war centuries in the future would exhibit convenient symptomatology that would arouse great suspicion, even disbelief, among those around them. Surely they were malingering, or making things up; they were really cowards who had lost the will to fight, and who sought to use mutism, tremors, sudden claims of blindness, or paralysis as excuses to avoid doing their duty. Yet these men, too, when subjected to creative, painful and sadistic treatments designed to flush out their fakery, would endure and persistently present their dubious deficits.

Still, hysterical men would be the exception, not nearly as rare as is often believed, to be sure, and certainly existing in defiance of one very common view of the disorder, that it was rooted in the female reproductive organs, more specifically, the womb (whether wandering or otherwise)—as its very name, deriving from the Greek word for that organ, *hystera*, would imply. More commonly, though, the hysterical patient would turn out to be female, and such remain the common-sense associations the word "hysteria" conjures up, in an age when professional psychiatrists have essentially abandoned the diagnosis. So here, too, Mary Glover is in some ways the prototypical hysterical patient, young and, more especially, female (though possibly a little *too* young for many, since she menstruated for the first time some months after the whole episode began). Gender plays a large and complex role in the biography of hysteria, so it is perhaps fitting that the first prominent English patient to be considered a hysteric should be a young unmarried girl.

And what of religion, that competing explanation of the London teenager's fits? That too will resurface as part of the biography of this baffling, recalcitrant, protean disorder, though, like Marx's Hegel, it will, in the process, be turned upside down. If the divine and the diabolical had once been invoked to account for hysterical symptoms and their cure, in centuries to come, in a secular not spirit-drenched world, hysteria would be a label put forth to explain away and discredit extreme varieties of the religious experience—the trances, the fugue states, the physical endurance, and the willingness to suffer of those Christians whom earlier generations of their co-religionists preferred to regard as saints.

II

NEUROLOGIE

As he began to lose his wits for the first time in 1788, George III announced to all who would listen that "I'm nervous, I'm not ill, but I'm nervous; if you would know what is the matter with me, I am nervous."[1] Sadly for him, the court and his physicians did not agree. Mad they called him, and soon he was being bled, blistered, starved, vomited, and purged, tied to his chair, menaced, placed in a strait waistcoat, whipped, and cut off from all contact with the outside world. Modern historians have broadly embraced the idea that his hallucinations, delusions, and delirious ravings were in all probability the side effects of an inherited metabolic disorder, porphyria, a disease that, appropriately enough, turned his urine purple. And certainly the king was far too disturbed ever to have been considered merely hysterical. But his embrace of the language of nervousness mirrored that of his subjects, among whom disordered nerves were now the *maladie à la mode*. A way of conceptualizing disease that would have made no sense even to most of the learned a century earlier had become common currency, embraced enthusiastically by the polite and *hoi polloi* alike. And occupying a central place among these "nervous disorders"

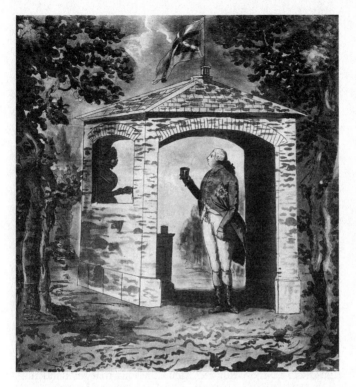

2. George III taking the waters at Cheltenham. Water cures were long a fashionable remedy for "nervous" complaints. (*Wellcome Library, London*)

was a complex of disturbances variously referred to as hysteria, hypochondria, the vapors, and the spleen.

Hysteria's migration from the uterine origins accorded it in Hippocratic and Galenic medicine to its new incarnation as a nervous complaint had begun to take place in the last third of the seventeenth century. The changed view of its etiology owed much, in the first instance, to the researches and writings of the royalist Sedleian Professor of Natural Philosophy at Oxford University, Thomas Willis, and to the subsequent pronouncements of his Puritan contemporary and rival Thomas Sydenham—famous for his emphasis on bedside observation rather than on books, and the physician often called the "English Hippocrates." Alongside, and to some extent instead of, the ancient Hippocratic notions of disease as a systemic disturbance of the four humors—blood, phlegm, black and yellow bile—these pre-eminent physicians began to explore an alternative system of bodily regulation, the nervous system, as a new source of disequilibrium and debility. In some respects, these ideas were obviously at odds with tradition, and yet the nerves were, like the circulation of the blood, something that could be incorporated into the more broadly based model of illness that was almost universally embraced at the time.

Disease of all sorts, for seventeenth- and eighteenth-century Englishmen, was constitutional, a symptom of an underlying disorder of the body that was systemic in nature. What surfaced locally as symptoms was often just the manifestation of the deep-seated disturbance of the body's equilibrium, and just how that disturbance manifested itself was in turn dependent upon one's inheritance and circumstances. Hence the notion of disease specificity was discounted. It followed as well that not just hysteria but other diseases were malleable and mobile, capable of migrating to different parts of the body as they developed, and mutating into different (and potentially more dangerous) disorders. Treatment in consequence was often a matter of getting disease out of the body, via purges and vomits and bleedings, through measures designed to sweat it out, or through counter-irritation designed to draw the disease away from the most dangerous areas of the human frame, and provide a route out of the system—blisters, issues, setons, and so forth.

In the years after Charles II's restoration to the throne in 1660, Thomas Willis undertook a sustained effort to understand the anatomy of the brain and the central nervous system. Though a technician, Richard Lower, did much of the actual work of dissection, Willis's theorizing based on these observations formed the foundation of a thoroughgoing reassessment of the nature and role of the nervous system in animating the human body.

> The anatomy of the nerves [nervous system], [he proclaimed in 1664], provides more pleasant and profitable speculations than the theory concerning any other part of the animal body: for by means of it, are revealed the true and genuine reasons for very many of the actions and passions that take place in our body, which otherwise seem most difficult to explain: and from this fountain, no less than the hidden cases of diseases and symptoms, which are commonly ascribed to the incantations of witches, may be discovered and satisfactorily explained.[2]

Mind and body met and somehow interacted in and through the brain and the nervous system, and the "animal spirits" that Willis viewed as commanding and controlling the body were powerful agents whose derangement could be invoked to explain all manner of illness and pathology. Here was a new arena for medicine that he dubbed "neurologie," one concerned with what many came to see as "the first" or the most "noble" of the body's organs.

A man of modest origins, Willis was plain in appearance and manner, and afflicted with a stammer, but he was, in seventeenth-century parlance, a skilled natural philosopher. He had been marginalized by his royalist sympathies during the time of Cromwell, and his initial forays into clinical practice brought him only a modicum of success. The sort of moneyed and titled clientele who patronized the most prominent gentlemanly physicians largely eluded him, and as a practitioner he had to make do with an itinerant practice in the market towns in the Oxford area. For several years, even following the Restoration, he occupied much of his time with the experimental examination of the brain and the nerves, and their presumed connections to sensation, motivation, thought, and behavior, topics on which he began to publish extensively in Latin in the 1660s, shortly before he moved to London. His anatomical drawings were concrete illustrations of his radically different conception of the brain, for his use of preservatives allowed him to see the organ as no one had before him. Folds and fissures, the distinction between a variety of distinct regions and features of the brain—the brain stem, the pons, the medulla, and the circle of arteries at the base of the brain (still known as the circle of Willis)—the visualization of the infolding of the cerebellum and cerebral cortex, the structures of the mid-brain, all these marked a dramatic reconceptualization of the physical reality of the brain, and of its role as the organ of thought.

Willis's relocation to the metropolis in 1667 proved to be a great success. The erudite if unprepossessing medical man rather belatedly acquired an enviable practice among the fashionable and socially prominent, and, following his death, his writings were soon translated into the vernacular, accelerating the circulation of his somewhat radical ideas about the sources of diseases in general, and of convulsive disorders in particular. Among these Willis numbered, not just epilepsy or the falling sickness, but a cluster of disorders involving the hysterical passions and the hypochondriacal affections.

The pathologies that produced hysteria and analogous disorders were, he asserted, firmly rooted in "the Brain and the

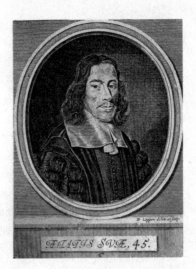

3. Thomas Willis (1621–75),
coiner of the term "neurologie,"
and Sedleian Professor of Natural
Philosophy at Oxford University.
(*Wellcome Library, London*)

Nervous Stock." They involved disturbances of sensation, motion, and consciousness that fell short of the "universal Convulsions" that marked true epilepsy, but were a closely related family of diseases. (The eminent nineteenth-century French neurologist Jean-Martin Charcot was of similar mind, often referring to "hystero-epilepsy.") It was "some taint" of the animal spirits "possessing the beginning of the Nerves within the head" that was productive of the disorder, "and whatever inordination, or irregularity from thence happens...is only secondary."[3]

Willis was well aware that, in making these claims, he was taking issue with the received wisdom about hysteria that had lasted for millennia. This "half damn'd" disorder was, he acknowledged, one of

> so ill fame, among the Diseases belonging to women, that...it bears the faults of many other Distempers: For

> when at any time, a sickness happens in a woman's body, of an unusual manner, or more occult original, so that its Cause lyes hid, and the Curatory Indication is altogether uncertain, presently we accuse the evill influence of the womb...and in every unusual Symptom, we declare it to be something hysterical.

Wide was the range of symptoms attributed to this distemper:

> A motion in the bottom of the belly, and an ascension of the same, as it were a certain round thing, then a belching, or a striving to vomit, a distention, and murmur of the hypochondria, with a breaking forth of blasts of winde, an unequall breathing and very much hindered, a choaking in the throat, a vertigo, an inversion, or rolling about of the eyes, oftentimes laughing, or weeping, absurd talking, sometimes want of speech, and motionless, with an obscure or no pulse, and deadish aspect, sometimes Convulsive motions, in the face and Limbs, and sometimes in the whole body, are excited: but universal Convulsions rarely happen, and not unless this disease be in the very worst state...I have observed these Symptoms in maids before ripe age [puberty], also in old women after their flowers have left them; yea, sometimes the same kinde of Passions infest men...[4]

Here were a number of further departures from tradition. Hippocratic and Galenic texts had placed the uterus at the heart of many disorders suffered by the female half of humanity, unambiguously so in those labelled hysterical. "Most ancient, and indeed Modern Physitians," Willis acknowledged dryly, "refer them to the ascent of the womb, and vapours elevated from it." Not a quarter century before, in 1651, the great William Harvey, renowned for discovering the circulation of the blood, had given new voice to the ancient consensus. Hysteria was a female malady, perhaps the quintessential female malady.

> For the uterus is a most important organ, and brings the
> whole body to sympathize with it...When the uterus either
> rises up or falls down, or is in any way put out of place or
> is seized with spasm—how dreadful, then, are the mental
> aberrations, the delirium, the melancholy, the paroxysms of
> frenzy, as if the affected person were under the domination
> of spells, and all arising from unnatural states of the uterus.[5]

Willis would have none of it.

> The former opinion, although it plead antiquity, seems the
> less probable, for that the body of the womb is of so small a
> bulk, in virgins, and widdows, and is so strictly tyed by the
> neighbouring parts round about, that it cannot of it self be
> moved, or ascend from its place, nor could its motion be felt,
> if there were any: as to that vulgar opinion, or Reason taken
> from the vapours, we have often rejected it as wholly vain,
> and light...[6]

That the wandering womb of Antiquity was an anatomical
impossibility would be confirmed by the great eighteenth-
century Italian physician Giovanni Battista Morgagni (1682–1771),
author of the classic *The Seats and Causes of Diseases Investigated
by Anatomy* (1761). Morgagni's published work was the fruit of
six decades of labor, and he lent his considerable authority in
support of Willis's conclusion that in cases of hysteria and
hypochondria "the chief disorder is in the nervous system, as it
is called."[7] By the middle of the eighteenth century, though, the
once heretical idea had become a commonplace.

That shift had occurred in part because Willis's views on
nervous disorders were broadly shared by his great Puritan
contemporary and rival, Thomas Sydenham (though the latter
was neither interested himself in brain anatomy, nor saw it as
having any clinical relevance). Sydenham was convinced that

"no chronic disease occurs so frequently as this." As much as a sixth of his clientele, he announced, were of the hysterical persuasion, victims of "a farrago of disorderly and irregular phenomena." For him, this occasioned no surprise, "for few women (which sex [as he slyly noted] makes one half of the grown persons), excepting such as work and fare hardly, are quite free from every species of this disorder." And not just women deserved the diagnosis: "several men also, who lead a sedentary life and study hard, are afflicted with the same." To be sure, the men's complaints not infrequently acquired a different label: "yet upon comparing the hypochondriac complaints, which we judge to rise from obstructions of the spleen and other viscera, with these symptoms, which seize hysteric women, we find a great similitude between them." Indeed, "hypochondriasis (which we impute to some obstruction of the spleen or viscera) is as like [hysteria] as one egg is to another." Wild and unintelligible talk, terrible convulsions, vomiting, a sensation of choking, violent pain and palpitations of the heart, and an "even more disordered" state of the mind merely hinted at the diversity of shapes and forms hysteria might take. For "this disease is not more remarkable for its frequency, than for the numerous forms under which it appears, resembling most of the distempers wherewith mankind are afflicted." It might manifest itself in any region of the body, and, wherever it surfaced, "it immediately produces such symptoms as are peculiar thereto; so that unless the physician be a person of judgment and penetration he will be mistaken, and suppose such symptoms to arise from some essential disease of this or that particular part, and not from the *hysterical passion*."[8]

Sydenham's conception of hysteria differed from Willis's in some important respects. It was not fits as such that were central to his view of the disorder (though he acknowledged that "sometimes it causes terrible convulsions"), but rather that the symptoms these patients presented "cannot be accounted for on the common principle of investigating diseases ..." and surfaced in those who had a prior history of "disturbances of the mind, which are the usual causes of this disease." Willis had distanced himself from the psychological, employing a reductionist physiology to explain disorders of the nerves. Sydenham, by contrast, noted the frequent complication of depressive symptoms in patients presenting with "hysterical [or] hypochondriacal complaints." He insisted that

> their misfortune does not only proceed from a great indisposition of the body, for the *mind* is still more disordered, it being in the nature of this disease to be attended with an incurable despair; so that they cannot bear with patience to be told that there is hope of their recovery, easily imagining that they are liable to all the miseries that can befall mankind; and presaging the worst evils to themselves.

The passions—"grief ... terror, anger, distrust, and other hateful passions"—were both crucial to the genesis of hysteria, and central elements in its course. And many of its sufferers exhibited an extraordinary emotional lability: "All is caprice. They love without measure those whom they will soon hate without reason."[9] Yet none of these characteristics should come as a surprise, since, in crucial ways (ways that remained opaque and hard to specify), the nervous system was coming to be seen as the interface between the material and the psychic realms.

Seventeenth- and eighteenth-century physicians rarely laid hands on their patients, relying on head, not hand, as the basis of their diagnostic acumen, and leaving the stigmatizing manual tasks that were a necessary part of any direct examination of the patient's body to the lower-status surgeons. Inevitably, this neglect of the physical examination led to all manner of diagnostic errors. Most famously, a whole array of fashionable physicians in the spa town of Bath misdiagnosed David Hume's illness, assuring the eminent philosopher that his "bilious" complaints were eminently curable, and would lend themselves to cure by changed diet and regimen, and by drinking the foul, sulfurous, waters. And they were not the least discombobulated when the pre-eminent British surgeon John Hunter *did* venture to palpate Hume's abdomen and distinctly felt the cancerous liver tumor that would rapidly kill its possessor. In any event, all practitioners in the Augustan Age obviously lacked access to the sorts of diagnostic technology critical to the differentiation of diseases today. Thus such labels as "hysteria" and "hypochondria," which admittedly were protean categories embracing disorders that mimicked other forms of disease, must necessarily have caught in their net numerous afflictions that today would be assigned to a wholly different realm of neurological pathology—a fact that should remind us of the dangers and difficulties of retrospective diagnosis, and of the foolishness of assuming that, just because the label "hysteria" has survived across the centuries, its content has remained similarly unchanged. Undoubtedly, some of the people whom seventeenth- and eighteenth-century physicians diagnosed as hysterical would today be seen as suffering from some form of epilepsy, from multiple sclerosis or the effects of tertiary syphilis, or from malignant tumors that manifested themselves in mysterious bodily ailments. But the issue of "mistakes" in the diagnostic process cuts both ways. Still other seventeenth- and eighteenth-century patients, as Sydenham reminds us, were *not* diagnosed as cases of hysteria, when, in the hands of a different doctor, or at a different time, they most certainly would have been.

In its new "nervous" guise, hysteria (along with the vapors, hypochondria, and the spleen—labels that came to be used more or less interchangeably) incorporated the milder forms of another traditional mental disorder, melancholy. In humoral medicine, the origins of hypochondria had lain in an excess of black bile, which was thought to originate in the spleen. Hence the equivalence of those two terms. The fumes from the excessive bile were thought to ascend to the head, thereby creating cognitive and emotional disarray. More and more, however, these congeries of diseases were set apart from the various forms of Bedlam madness. Whether one looks to the social location of the sufferers, the treatment to be meted out to them, or their prospects of cure, in all these respects "nervous" patients were increasingly regarded very differently from those suffering from other forms of alienation.

Mania, dementia, and the darker forms of melancholia—those disturbances of the psyche that were often collectively referred to as lunacy or insanity—were not just signs of a far more serious complex of disorders, but occupied a different ontological status. Deprived of "the sovereign power of the soul" and the central defining characteristic of the human, Reason, the victims of out-and-out madness were dragged down into a state of brutish insensibility and incapacity. The veneer of civilization was stripped away, replaced by extravagance, incoherence, incomprehensibility, menace, rage, and unpredictable outbreaks of violence that revealed the beast within. In the words of the early eighteenth-century physician Nicholas Robinson, they were "the most gloomy Scene of Nature, that Mankind can possibly encounter... almost debas'd below the brutal Species of the animated Creation."[10] Their ferocity, as Thomas Willis had urged a half century earlier, could be tamed only by a mixture of discipline and depletion, measures designed to put down "the raging of the Spirits and the lifting up of the Soul." Even still, such creatures were scarcely within the reach of orthodox medical remedies, and instead required forceful, even violent, interventions, measures designed to induce "their reverence or standing in awe of such as they think their Tormentors." For in truth, "Furious Mad-men are sooner and more certainly cured by punishments and hard usage, in a strait-room, than by *Physick* or Medicines."[11]

Hysteria was different, persistent, but treatable with the standard remedies of antiphlogistic medicine: attention to diet and regimen, regulation of the body's evacuations, bleedings, purges, and vomits. Its victims, Willis acknowledged, "are healed more often with flatteries, and with more gentle Physick."[12] His efforts, and those of Sydenham, to link the disorder to the nerves had not at first drawn universal approbation or even much attention beyond the ranks of a handful of elite physicians. Katherine Williams's study of seventeenth-century manuscripts—doctors' private notebooks as well as the recipes for treating disease put together by womenfolk—has documented the persistence of traditional notions of hysteria's gynecological origins even as these high-status metropolitan physicians dismissed them as nonsensical. But, in the first third of the new century, among an increasing number of medical men and, at least as significantly, among the affluent classes to whom they sought to minister, the notion of hysteria's nervous etiology made major inroads.

In professional circles, the appeal of theories of nervousness derived in part from the more general rise in the popularity of applying mechanistic explanations to medical phenomena. Most obviously, this move towards what is often termed "iatromechanical" medicine derived from the general cultural prestige of the new Newtonian science. Accounts pitched in mechanistic terms, and invoking physical laws and processes (or sometimes chemical principles and knowledge), proliferated in the early eighteenth century and became a touchstone for the explanation of all sorts of bodily disorders. Through the efforts of Willis's and Sydenham's students and successors, enthusiastically taken up by a lay audience, the new notions of "animal spirits" moving speedily or slowly through the delicate network of tubes or fibres that made up the brain and nervous system soon achieved a wide currency.

Certainly, nerves were not the only possible physical culprit in cases of hysteria and hypochondria. The London physician John Purcell (1674–1730) thought that the underlying problem lay, not in the nervous system, but "in the *Stomach* and *Guts*; whereof the Grumbling of the one and the Heaviness and uneasiness of the other generally preceding the Paroxysm, in no small Proofs." "Vapours" from these regions, rising "up to the Head" produced the characteristic "Hysterick Fits... a Disease which more generally afflicts Humane Kind, than any other whatsoever; and Proteus-like, transforms it self into the shape and representation of almost all distempers..."[13] But many of his colleagues preferred to follow their eminent seventeenth-century predecessors and implicate the nervous system. John Pechey's *General Treatise of the Diseases of Maids, Big-Bellied Women, Childbed Women and Widows* appeared in 1698, and largely contented itself with paraphrasing Sydenham. Just over a decade later, Bernard Mandeville put related ideas into general circulation, couching his discussion of "the Hypochondriack and Hysterick Passions vulgarly call'd the Hypo in Men and the Vapours in Women" in the form of a dialogue between Philopirio, the doctor, and

Misombedon, the father of the patient, a literary device he self-consciously deployed "by way of [providing] Information to Patients" rather than "to teach other Practitioners."[14] And both the prominent metropolitan physician Sir Richard Blackmore and Nicholas Robinson, one of the governors of London's oldest madhouse, Bedlam, lent their authority to the cause.

Robinson, probably the most crudely reductionist of the lot, sought to account "mechanically" for all sorts of "Alterations of the Mind." Whether simple "Lownesses of the Spirits" or outright "Madness, and Lunacy," the origins of the mental disturbance was to be sought in "Changes in the Motion of the [nervous] Fibres." Others, he observed scornfully, were "ready to resolve all into Whim, or a wrong Turn of the Fancy." He emphatically did not share their erroneous views. "I deny," he insisted, with characteristic truculence,

> that all the Thoughts themselves can ever start from a regular Way of Thinking, without inferring, at the same Time, a Change in the Motions of the Animal Fibres…it's impossible that the Mind can suffer and the Body be unaffected at the same Time…Every Change of the Mind, therefore, indicates a Change in the bodily Organs; nor is it possible for the Wit of Man to conceive how the Mind can, from a chearful, gay Disposition, fall into a sad and disconsolate State, without some Alterations in the Fibres, at the same Time.[15]

Like others who seek to render mental faculties epiphenomenal (whether in the eighteenth century or now), Robinson was oblivious to the contradiction implicit in his decision to try to persuade others of the rightness of his views, whether by constant reiteration of his position, or by reasoned argument. "It clearly appears," he kept insisting, that whenever the Mind perceives itself uneasy, low-spirited, or dejected, it is as full a Demonstration, as the Nature of the Thing will admit, that the Instruments, by which the Mind directs the Powers of its Operations, are affected ... While the Nerves ... are in good Plight, the Ideas they convey through any of the Senses will be regular, just, and clear; upon which the Understanding will judge and determine of Objects, as they are, but the Laws of Nature ... But if the Structure or Mechanism of these Organs happen to be disorder'd, and the Springs of the Machine out of Tune; no Wonder the Mind perceives the Alteration, and is affected with the Change.[16]

If hysteria was a symptom of a "machine out of tune," and, more ominously, a disorder that in Robinson's view differed in degree but not in kind from madness itself, it nonetheless (like its twin hypochondria) was emphatically a genuine disease. All these forms of mental alienation, "from the slightest Symptoms of the Spleen and Vapours, to the most confirm'd Affections of Melancholy Madness and Lunacy ... are no imaginary Whims or Fancies, but real Affections of the Mind, arising from the real, mechanical Affections of Matter and Motion, whenever the Constitution of the Brain warps from its natural Standard." Hence, "compleating a successful Cure" depended upon employing medical remedies, even "Medicines of the Brain, necessary to procure a Freedom from those Affections, the Mind labours under during the Continuance of this Disease."[17] On the central claim that hysteria was a real disease, Robinson was as one with other leading society physicians, even those who adopted a more nuanced view of mind–body interactions and who embraced milder modes of treatment.

Sir Richard Blackmore, for example, who had served as William III's and Queen Anne's personal physician, was equally emphatic that hysteria belonged in the medical man's province, and that it shaded imperceptibly into "Melancholy, Lunacy, and Phrenzy." Like Sydenham and Willis before him, Blackmore insisted that, though others tried to distinguish them, in essence hysteria and hypochondria were

> the same malady…It is true that the convulsive Disorders and Agitations in the various Parts of the Body, as well as the Confusion and Dissipation of the animal Spirits, are more conspicuous and violent in the Female Sex, than in Men; the Reason of which is, a more volatile, dissipable, and weak Constitution of the Spirits, and a more soft, tender, and delicate Texture of the Nerves [among women]; but this proves no Difference in their Nature and essential Properties, but only a higher or lower degree of the symptoms common to both.[18]

Blackmore acknowledged, however, that "This Disease, called Vapours in Women, and the Spleen in Men, is what neither Sex are pleased to own." Speaking one suspects from personal experience, he lamented that a physician "cannot ordinarily make his Court [his chances of obtaining fees from a moneyed patient] worse, than by suggesting to such Patients the true Nature and Name of their Distemper."[19] A major reason for the patients' reluctance to accept the diagnosis was, he was convinced, that those who had never suffered from it dismissed it as a purely imaginary disorder, and hysterics thus felt themselves subject to derision and contempt. But, even if the disease was the product of "fancy" and imagination, the pains they suffered were real and unfeigned. Terrible ideas, all by themselves, could produce pain in both brain and body.

With respect to therapeutics, Sir Richard was one of those who took strong issue with Robinson's advocacy of "the most violent Vomits, the strongest purging Medicines, and large Bleeding…often repeated" as the appropriate treatment for hysteria.[20] Patients suffering from the disease, Blackmore insisted, were often afflicted with great despondency and anxiety, for which the best response was calming prescriptions. It did no good to assault the patient with fearsome and painful remedies. On the contrary, strong purges and the like would only enfeeble the system and ultimately undermine and "demolish" the patient. He should rather be composed and strengthened, and perhaps calmed with opium, thus strengthening his system and restoring him to health.

Save for masochists, and those sad souls convinced that, unless treatments were painful and unpleasant they were unlikely to do much good, such milder prescriptions were probably the more popular among prospective patients, and the need to attract patients was, of course, of paramount importance to all these practitioners. Physicians' books and treatises, though ostensibly aimed to some extent at their professional brethren, were simultaneously a way of raising their profile among an affluent and educated lay audience, who, for much of the eighteenth century, shared a common set of cultural assumptions about illness and its treatment with their doctors, and expected to play an active role in the encounter with those they regarded (quite correctly by the standards of their time) as their social inferiors. In a period of growing affluence, one that saw the birth of what historians have dubbed the first consumer society, the market for all sorts of consumer goods and services was expanding apace, and, like other entrepreneurs, those who portrayed themselves as the purveyors of health and long life sought every opportunity to expand their customer base. Expanding public awareness of hysteria and related disorders, and laying claim to expertise in managing these illnesses, were obvious strategies for physicians to pursue, promising access to a far more fashionable and desirable clientele than the Bedlam mad. Here, indeed, was an extraordinarily attractive patient population, blessed with excessively refined sensibilities and exquisitely civilized temperaments (not to mention money).

What these medical men may not have fully realized, however, was just how attractive their assertions that hysteria was a physical disease like any other, a genuine disorder of the nerves, would prove to be among the moneyed and the fashionable crowd. Not for the last time in hysteria's history, it turned out that prospective patients were hungry for reassurance that their pain and suffering were real, just like other forms of illness, and that they deserved the dignity of the sick role, not the opprobrium that accrues to counterfeiters and frauds. (When John Radcliffe had ventured to suggest that his royal patient Queen Anne was suffering from the vapors, which she regarded as suggesting her pains were imaginary or doubtful, she promptly fired him.) So the notion that the rise of "nervous" disorders was simply the invention of the self-interested professionals requires some balance. If the profession was eager, whole segments of the population they sought to serve turned out to be every bit as willing to embrace their new-fangled ideas.

III

AN ENGLISH MALADY?

George Cheyne was a Scottish physician, one of a parade of ambitious and talented young men who had moved south to make their fortune around the time of the 1707 Act of Union between the two kingdoms of England and Scotland. A wit and initially something of a wastrel, Cheyne had sought to build his practice among the socially superior by hanging around the London coffee houses, flattering his would-be customers, polishing his credentials as a modern follower of Newtonian notions, and eating and drinking himself to a gargantuan size. More than 32 stone, or almost 450 pounds at his peak fighting weight, Cheyne grew so corpulent that he could barely move, and so naturally set himself up as a diet doctor. Affluence and luxury, after all, set loose the appetites, and excess exacts a predictable price in expanding waistlines and that quintessential eighteenth-century disease, gout. Who was better placed to preach restraint than one who had experienced at first hand the perils of its opposite?

But Cheyne was also a man prone to bouts of depression and despair, blessed or cursed with the very sort of nervous temperament that his professional brethren were now making so much

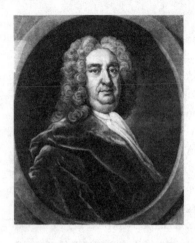

4. George Cheyne (1671–1743) in 1732, a year before the appearance of *The English Malady*—a picture that flatters the corpulent diet doctor. (*Wellcome Library, London*)

of. One is tempted to suggest that he leapt on the bandwagon, but leaping was, of course, not an activity George was actually able to perform. (By the late 1710s, forced to support his almost unsupportable bulk, his legs "broke out all over in scorbutick ulcers" and he confessed that, "if I had but an hundred paces to walk, I was oblig'd to have a servant following me with a Stool to sit on."[1]) His own mental anguish, however, had brought him to a certain sympathy with the hysteric and the hypochondriac, and his trolling for suitably affluent patients had already secured him at least one well-connected "nervous" patient, Catherine Walpole, the oldest daughter of the Whig grandee and prime minister, Sir Robert Walpole, whose patronage Cheyne secured courtesy of the far more established physician to the aristocracy, Sir Hans Sloane.

Catherine became Cheyne's patient in April 1720. Just 16, the young woman had come to Bath, like many of the *jeunesse dorée* of her generation, to partake of the waters, a remedy increasingly embraced by the leisured classes. But Catherine's symptoms seemed more serious than most. She displayed an alarming lack of appetite, a propensity to vomit, and complained of mysterious pains in her side. Then there were "fitts" and faintings, mysterious swellings, and amenorrhea (quite possibly the result of malnutrition). "It was rumoured," as Cheyne wrote to Sloane, that "disappointments [in love] had some hand in [her] original ail."[2] In time-honored fashion, the doctor sought to regulate the equilibrium of her system by encouraging her evacuations and the restoration of her menses, "wherein, I take a good deal of her Distemper to Ly." (The excess of retained blood, he thought, found its way to the brain, and there prompted her hysteria.) Spa waters were observed to have a cathartic effect, and to these Cheyne added such purgatives as rhubarb, castor oil, and a bitter emmenagogue, together with lavender to strengthen her nerves.

Catherine's mother appears to have been less than impressed than her husband with her daughter's Scottish physician, and sought a second opinion from a more experienced rival, Sir David Hamilton. Professional courtesy prevailed, however, and Hamilton largely endorsed Cheyne's prescriptions. At length, there appeared to be some progress—at least, Catherine began to menstruate. But her pains and debility continued, and Sir Robert wrote to Cheyne in the summer of 1720, lamenting: "Her severall symptoms are worse rather than better." The patient herself insisted on moving from Bristol (whose cooling waters Cheyne had recommended) back to Bath, where he found her prone to repeated fainting fits, constipated by the opiates she had been taking, and convinced that she would have died had she stayed on in Bristol. By October, she seemed much better. Cheyne boasted: "She has had none of the Great fitts (which

I call Hysterick) these 12 or 14 days. Her faintings are less frequent…[her] only Complaint…is her sickness after eating, which indeed is terrible…" A month later, bathing in the Bath waters had brought further improvement, and she was seen as "most miraculously recovered," so much so that she promptly left for London for the "season" of dinners and balls that marked the coming of age of a young aristocratic lady.

Soon, however, Catherine entered a slow decline. Cheyne prescribed mercurial purgatives (which seems an odd choice of medicine for one so frail and inclined to vomit up her food), and combined these with a new course of Bath waters. Many of her more prominent symptoms seemed to abate, but he fretted nonetheless that she "lives all most on air and water, two thin Elements; she eats not food Sufficient to Maintain a Parrot." Catherine grew emaciated. Her legs swelled. She became "totally obstructed." Recognizing that she had "but faint hopes of…Recovery," Cheyne first redoubled her purgatives, and then in despair indicated that he planned "to let her do just as she pleases, to attempt nothing… & wait till Nature has releas'd her, or indicated some thing that may effectually relieve her." Nature apparently declined to indicate a way forward, and 18-year-old Catherine soon succumbed, dying at Bath in early October 1722, just a little more than two years after Cheyne had been summoned to her bedside.

So pronounced and public a failure with so prominent a patient might have been expected to inflict grave damage on Cheyne's professional prospects. Not a bit of it. Cheyne was helped, of course, by the fact that patients and their families had lower expectations for medicine's powers in the early eighteenth century. But his continued success had other sources as well, for the good doctor had discovered he had an unequaled talent for writing medical treatises aimed at a general audience. Writing popular books on gout, and on diet as the royal road to health and longevity, propelled Cheyne to an ever greater prominence over the next decade. When combined with his obsequious deference to his social superiors (in full view in his surviving correspondence with one of his more prominent "hysterical" patients, the Countess of Huntingdon), it brought him an ever larger clientele among the affluent and the nervous. Seizing the opportunity, Cheyne capitalized on his reputation to expand his practice to a quite remarkable extent.

Just as syphilis had been variously labeled the French disease (by the English), the Spanish disease (by the French), and the Neapolitan disease (by the Spanish), no one wanting to own so stigmatizing a disorder, so Europeans had been pleased to poke fun at the English as peculiarly prone to melancholy and what were by now seen increasingly as nervous disorders. Blackmore had glumly noted that one synonym for the "hysterical affections" was "the English spleen; since it has here gained such a universal and tyrannical Dominion over both Sexes, as incomparably exceeds its Power in other Nations..."[3] It was Cheyne's conceit to turn this reproach into an occasion for celebrating England's national superiority, a superiority that then, as now, seemed self-evident to his fellow countrymen.

The English Malady, the most popular of all Cheyne's guides to health, appeared in 1733, and only two years later was already in its sixth edition. In its pages, Cheyne loudly proclaimed that "nervous Disorders...a Class and Set of Distempers, with atrocious and frightful Symptoms, scarce known to our Ancestors," were responsible for "almost one third of the Complaints" of the age.[4] They were a commonplace—or at least, as he hastened to add, were a commonplace among "the People of Condition in England." For the various manifestations "of nervous diseases of all kinds, as Spleen, Vapours, Hypochondriacal and Hysterical Distempers" were the unlucky province of the social elite: the urbane, the cultivated, the refined, the delicate. Sensibility, after all, was a quality of the civilized—indeed of the quality. It was absent among *hoi polloi*, for the lower orders were like wood, dull, essentially unfeeling creatures, and "Fools, weak or stupid Persons, heavy and dull Souls, are seldom troubled with Vapours or Lowness of Spirits"—any more than is "a heavy, dull, earthy, clod-pated Clown."[5] By contrast, the more refined, delicate nervous systems of the elite put them at risk of falling into hysterics and related nervous states, for it was those "of the liveliest and quickest natural Parts, whose Faculties are the most bright and spiritual, whose Genius is most keen and penetrating, and particularly where there is the most delicate Sensation and Taste,"[6] who were most prone to such disorders. (No wonder that Cheyne was proud to boast that he ranked among their number, his own case being presented "at large" (*sic*—Cheyne was deaf to irony) in the book's closing pages.)

Nervous diseases, hysteria most notably among them, were diseases of civilization. Their extraordinary proliferation in the higher ranks of English society, so far from being a reproach, was a sign of England's global superiority over all its rivals. Among primitive peoples, "Temperance, Exercise, Hunting, Labour, and Industry kept the Juices sweet, and the Solids brac'd." Where all was "simple, plain, honest, and frugal, there were few or no diseases."[7] But in modern times, the ambition for success in business brought "Anxiety and Concern." Its achievement led to diversions and dissipation. Both betrayed the nerves, and brought with them suffering and prostration.

It was England's unbridled success, the triumph of its economic and social arrangements, that made hysteria and associated nervous complaints so prominent a part of its medical landscape. "Since our Wealth has increas'd, and our Navigation has been extended, we have ransack'd all parts of the Globe to bring together its whole Stock of Materials for *Riot*, *Luxury*, and to provoke *Excess*...sufficient to provoke, and even gorge, the most large and voluptuous Appetite."[8] The English climate, "the Moisture of our Air, the Variableness of our Weather," did not help matters. But the true sources of England's unwanted preeminence in the realm of nervous disorders were "the Rankness and Fertility of our Soil, the Richness and Heaviness of our Food, the Wealth and Abundance of the Inhabitants (from their universal Trade), the Inactivity and sedentary Occupations of the better Sort (among whom this Evil mostly rages), and the Humour of living in great, populous and consequently unhealthy Towns..."[9] The "English malady," in other words, was in large measure a badge of honor, not of shame.

There was, to be sure, not just a perverse national pride, but also a scolding, puritanical tone to some of Cheyne's admonitions. "If *Nervous* Disorders are the Diseases of the Wealthy, the Voluptuous, and the Lazy," he lectured his audience, "and are mostly produc'd, and always aggravated and increased, by *Luxury* and *Intemperance*...there needs no great Depth of Penetration to find out that *Temperance* and *Abstinence* is necessary towards their Cure."[10] The rich were upbraided for their "Gluttony and Intemperance in fermented Liquors, and...unguarded Leachery," as well as other forms of "Excess." Indulging in the richest and strongest foods, cramming themselves with tea and coffee, chocolate and tobacco, they simply transgressed the rules of healthy lives. Besides, they lived an artificial and contrived urban existence, replete with luxury and temptation, and dominated by foolish fashion. Foreign delicacies, imported to stimulate their jaded palates, encouraged them to overeat, while their sedentary lives left them bereft of exercise and deprived of sleep. Small wonder so many of them fell victim to nervous complaints: convulsions, faintings, dislocated speech, despondency, screaming, silence, laughter, or tears without apparent cause.

A number of his colleagues had made much of the claim that hysteria was a real illness. Cheyne loudly endorsed their views, contending that "of all the Miseries that afflict Human Life, and relate principally to the Body, in this Valley of Tears, I think *Nervous* Disorders, in their extream and last Degrees, are the most deplorable, and beyond comparison the worst."[11] One of his most eminent colleagues had once confided to him that

> he had seen Persons labouring under the most exquisite Pains of Gout, Stone, Colick, Cancer, and all the other Distempers that can tear the human Machin, yet he had observed them all willing to prolong their wretched Being, and scarce any ready to lay down cheerfully the Load of Clay...but such as labour'd under a constant, internal Anxiety, meaning those most sinking, suffocating, and strangling Nervous Disorders.[12]

Yet the "Vulgar and Unlearned," Cheyne commented with some disdain, compounded the pain and suffering of the victims by placing "Nervous Distempers...under some Kind of Disgrace," regarding the condition either as "a lower Degree of Lunacy, and the first Step towards a distemper'd Brain"; or else as mere "Whim, Ill-Humour, Peevishness or Particularity; and in the [female] Sex, Daintiness, Fantasticalness, or Coquetry."[13] So widespread were these prejudices that Cheyne confessed that, in his own practice, frequently "I have been in the utmost Difficulty, when desir'd to define or name the Distemper, for fear of affronting them, or fixing a Reproach on a Family or Person."[14] Like Sir Richard Blackmore before him, Cheyne responded by insisting that the Brain was indeed involved, and not in any imaginary or metaphorical way: "the Disease," he pronounced authoritatively, "is as much a bodily Distemper...as the Small-Pox or a Fever."[15]

It was a viewpoint embraced enthusiastically by Cheyne's patients, whose circle had by now expanded to include a duke, a bishop and the Canon of Christ Church, and a litany of lords and ladies, from Lord Chesterfield to the Countess of Huntingdon. Not only were they reassured that their sufferings, which others cavalierly dismissed as *maladies imaginaires*, were as real, as rooted in the defects of the body, as any the skeptics might name, but their illness was even a mark of distinction, a badge of honor. No more laughing at their misery, no more dismissing them as frauds or fakes. It can be no coincidence that over the last decade of his life, as he reported to his friend and publisher, the novelist Samuel Richardson, Cheyne's income tripled, for his enormous financial success provided the most practical indication of the success of his ideas in the cultural marketplace. Insisting that their sufferings were organic and not their own invention, patients were as highly motivated as their entrepreneurial doctors to designate their disorders as genuine diseases.

The fashionability of hysteria and its cognates can as easily be traced in the persistent references to nervous complaints in contemporary novels, drama, and poetry. Umbriel's address to the Queen of Spleen in Alexander Pope's *The Rape of the Lock* provides just one example of a literary figure making fun of ladies affecting the "vapors" as a sign of superior sensibility:

Hail, wayward Queen!
Who rule the sex to fifty from fifteen:
Parent of vapours and of female wit,
Who give th' hysteric, or poetic fit,
On various tempers act by various ways,
Make some take physic, others scribble plays.

Meantime, even so pronounced a skeptic as the philosopher David Hume could be found echoing Cheyne, avowing in his *Treatise on Human Nature* (1739) that "the skin, pores, muscles, and nerves of a day-labourer are different from those of a man of quality so are his sentiments, actions and manners." Some years later, his fellow Scot James Boswell was so taken with the conceit that to be nervous was a mark of superior sensibility as to pen a whole series of autobiographical columns under the pseudonym "The Hypochondriack," boasting there that "we *Hypochondriacks* may console ourselves in the hour of gloomy distress, by thinking that our sufferings mark our superiority."[16] (Obviously he had not been deterred by Samuel Johnson's stern injunction to him: "Do not let [Cheyne] teach you a foolish notion that melancholy is a proof of acuteness."[17])

Dr Johnson was not alone in recoiling from the fashionable embrace of nervous disorders, the self-regarding and self-parodying culture where succumbing to sickness and morbid sensibilities became a matter of honor. Jonathan Swift prided himself on being "a perfect stranger to the spleen,"[18] and his fellow Tory, the perpetually unwell Alexander Pope, he who once referred to this "long Disease, my Life,"[19] nonetheless proclaimed on his deathbed, "I was never hyppish in my life."[20] However intent the hysterics and hypochondriacs were on securing validation of their illnesses from others, to put it mildly, not everyone was convinced that they had an organic illness, and were not malingering.

To be sure, the professional embrace of the nerves showed no signs of slackening. In the next generation, for instance, Robert Whytt, Professor of Medicine at Edinburgh, the leading center of medical learning in eighteenth-century Britain, devoted himself to the experimental study of the nervous system, and threw his prestige behind the idea that hysteria was indeed a disorder of the nerves. His skill at elucidating various properties of the nervous system, establishing, for instance, that nervous impulses could initiate movement independent of either the will or external stimuli (what he called "vital" and "involuntary motions," and later generations would call autonomic and reflex activity), lent an authority to his pronouncements about the nervous origins of hysteria and hypochondria that they scarcely merited. For Whytt in essence could do more than gesture at a rag-tag series of "causes" for these disorders: worms, blockages of the digestive viscera, phlegm, improper nourishment, a presumed uncommon weakness or delicacy of the nerves, or the impact of strong passions—"horrible or unexpected sights, great grief, anger, terror [occasioning] the most sudden and violent nervous symptoms"—any or all of these might "throw a person into hysteric fits, either of the convulsive or fainting kind."[21]

Whether the nervous system was conceived of as a network of hollow pipes, through which fluids flowed in a hydraulic system; or, as Cheyne suggested, as "Bundles of *solid, springy*, and *elastick* Threads or Filaments (like Twisted *Cat-Guts* or *Hairs*)";[22] or as a series of fibres or strings, it provided what Roy Porter has called an "alternative geography of anguish and action".[23] Often, that new geography placed the brain at the center of the story, but, as Whytt's reference to the digestive viscera indicates, this was not always the case. At the very end of the eighteenth century, William Heberden preferred to emphasize the sympathetic connections between guts and brain, and the role of the digestive system in the genesis and the treatment of hysteria: "The nerves of the stomach and bowels have so great a domain and controul over the whole nervous system, and these parts are so generally disordered in hypochondriac and hysteric patients, that, in my judgement, the best medicines will be such as correct their acidities."[24]

The very centrality of the nervous system in the regulation of all parts of the body (a centrality that would lead William Cullen, who was by common consent the most influential medical teacher at Edinburgh in the second half of the eighteenth century, to proclaim that "in a certain view, almost the whole of the diseases of the human body might be called *nervous*"[25]) meant that other geographies of hysteria might emerge in the light of its reclassification as a nervous disease (what Cullen had dubbed a "neurosis"). And so in the Victorian age it would prove. The protean reach and importance of the nerves meant something more: the proliferation of nervous complaints. At the dawn of a new century, Thomas Trotter proclaimed their unsettling triumph: "we do not hesitate to affirm that *nervous disorders*...may be justly reckoned, two thirds of the whole, with which civilized society is afflicted." Worse yet, "nervous ailments are no longer confined to the better ranks in life, but [are] rapidly extending to the poorer classes."[26]

From the very beginning, the emergence of a nervous etiology for hysteria had also raised the possibility of a new social geography for the disease. Hippocratic and Galenic theories, which had tied hysteria's etiology to the female reproductive system, had suggested that it was a disorder only of one half of the human species. Yet it had not entirely escaped notice that there were men who exhibited comparable symptoms. The new doctrine of the nerves made it easy to extend the diagnosis to males, and both Willis and Sydenham had explicitly recognized the existence of male hysterics. For all that, women were still seen as contributing a disproportionate share to the ranks of the sufferers, a disparity that seemed easy to explain, for the female frame, and the female nervous system, were simply a frailer, lest robust version of the male. Women's nerves were more delicate, their brains more susceptible to breakdown.

In Cheyne's version of the consensus, nervous disorders were associated with "weak, tender, and delicate Constitutions," whereas "those of large, full, and (as they are call'd) mastiff Muscles, and of big and strong Bones, are generally of a firmer State of Fibres"[27] (and thus unlikely to display the symptoms of hysteria). "Soft and yielding, loose and flabby Flesh and Muscles, are sure Symptoms of weak and relaxed Nerves or Fibres," as was "a fat, corpulent, and phlegmatic Constitution."[28] The gendered implications of such distinctions are clear, and yet, of course, the characteristics that revealed a predisposition to hysteria, while predominantly found among the female of the species, were by no means confined to that half of creation. But the males who shared these traits were, as was freely adumbrated in the literature, weak, effeminate creatures bereft of the qualities generally seen as appropriately masculine.

This sense of the hysterical male as somehow lacking, and the hint of homosexuality that lay mostly unspoken behind such portraits, was a trope that persisted well into the nineteenth century. Indeed, perhaps the quintessential rendering of the type was Wilkie Collins's memorable creation, the feckless Frederick Fairlie, a central figure in one of the most famous fictional renderings of madness, *The Woman in White*. Mr Fairlie is introduced to us

> dressed in a dark frock-coat, of some substance much thinner than cloth, and in waistcoat and trousers of spotless white. His feet were effeminately small, and were clad in buff-coloured silk stockings, and little womanish bronze-leather slippers. Two rings adorned his white delicate hands…Upon the whole he had a frail, languidly-fretful, over-refined look—something singularly and unpleasantly delicate in its association with a man, and, at the same time, something which could by no possibility have looked natural and appropriate if it had been transferred to the appearance of a woman.

Possessed of "a querulous, croaking voice," he is hypersensitive to light, noise, even the residual smells of the lower orders who may have handled his *objets d'art*, and incapable of enduring any sort of mental upset or strain without threatening to faint on the spot. Lest the reader miss the point, we observe him "leering at the cherubs" who appear in "his matchless Rembrandt etchings," and are informed by the family lawyer that "marrying and leaving an heir [were] the two very last things in the world he was likely to do." Put otherwise, in Frederick Fairlie's own words, we encounter "nothing but a bundle of nerves dressed up to look like a man…shattered…exhausted…prostrated," and, as we have a multitude of occasions to observe, selfish in the highest degree—thus the veritable archetype of the male hysteric.

For the most part, the embrace of the nervous theory of the origins of hysteria, while legitimizing the notion of the male hysteric, had little obvious impact on therapeutics. A stress on diet, sleep, and exercise, and on diverting the mind, coupled

with the standard remedies of traditional, antiphlogistic medicine—all this made for a therapeutic regime that differed little
from what might have been prescribed a century and more
earlier. Cheyne's prescription for his friend Samuel Richardson
was entirely typical:

> I hope your Case is more Hypochondriacal than Apoplectic.
> I am for losing a little Blood once in 2 or 3 months, taking a
> Vomit some days after, drinking only Valerian Small Beer and
> Valerian Tea [for their diuretic effects]—the more the better
> of either—living on half a Chicken in Quantity of any fresh
> tender Meat (any Things else to fill Chinks you please), and
> drinking only half a Pint of Wine with Water and Small Beer
> a Day, useing all the House or Abroad Exercise you can, keep-
> ing good Hours, and never applying [working] long at a time,
> and for Drugs only these [mercury] pills [to purge you].[29]

There was, however, one striking exception to this picture of
a changed intellectual account of the origins of hysteria married to therapeutic stasis. First in Hapsburg Vienna, and then,
when scandal threatened, in pre-Revolutionary Paris, a well-
to-do Austrian physician, Franz Anton Mesmer, modified the
doctrine of the nerves, and claimed to have discovered a new
active principle at work controlling the body: one that he had
mastered, and could use to dramatic effect. Employing his
innovation allowed the nervous to be restored to the ranks of
the hale and hearty.

In some mysterious fashion, there was broad agreement by
the last third of the eighteenth century that the nerves ministered between mind and brain, possessing some of the attributes
of both. They carried signals and messages to the brain, the
sensations on which that organ depended, and in the opposite
direction they carried its orders, and animated the machine

that was the human body. As for the means by which these signals and orders passed back and forth, a variety of models and
metaphors were posited. Some believed firmly in fibers, others
in fluids. Some spoke of a nervous ether, others of a nervous
electricity.

Mesmer claimed to have identified a different nerve force.
Having earlier tried electricity and steel magnets as curative instruments (a not uncommon tactic at the time), he had
observed, or so he thought, a related and more subtle power
bearing some similarities to these, but unique to the human
body, a property he began to refer to as animal magnetism.
Here was a natural healing power, a "fluidum," that provided a
means of influencing the nervous system and curing all manner of disease. Its strength could be augmented and directed, for
certain people (Mesmer himself, of course, prominent among
them) possessed the ability to harness this mysterious force,
even to transfer some of it from the outside into the body of the
patient. That might occur simply through the force of one's gaze,
or through the laying-on of hands, or even through "passes"
(the movement of the hands over the surface of the body without actually touching it). Or it could happen by sitting down at
a tub filled with iron filings, from which protruded rods that the
patients might grasp to access the stored magnetic energy.

Mesmer's most prominent patient in Vienna was an 18-year-
old blind pianist, Maria Theresia Paradis, who, as a result of his
attentions, announced that she could see. That those attentions
might have extended beyond the bounds of professional propri-
ety was only one of the rumors Mesmer's jealous competitors
circulated about him. Worse still, perhaps, Paradis discovered
that her recovery from her presumably hysterical blindness
was not exactly a useful professional move, as demand for her

concerts fell sharply once she could see. Not long afterwards, she announced she was blind again, a relapse seized upon by Mesmer's enemies. Within three months, he felt forced to flee the debacle, ending up in Paris.

Among the French aristocracy, especially the female aristocrats, Mesmer's reputation as a charismatic healer spread rapidly. His house in Paris was overwhelmed by crowds of the nervous and the hysterical, seeking relief from their troubles and pains. The baquet (a specially designed tub filled with animal magnetism, whose curative properties were transmitted to patients via the iron rods that protruded from it) allowed for treatment en masse, and Mesmer soon hypothesized that the passage of magnetic fluid to large numbers rather than a single patient augmented rather than reduced its therapeutic effects. To accentuate the effects of the treatment, soft music was added (Mesmer taking a turn on a glass harp, which he apparently played rather well), and the good doctor dressed in a lavender-colored silk robe, and wandered among his ecstatic patients, brushing them with a long magnetized iron rod. On occasion, he magnetized oak trees and streams, and removed the whole enterprise outdoors. His mostly female patients swooned and swore they were vastly improved, while Mesmer's professional rivals, seeing their wealthy patients flock to these séances, gnashed their teeth, spoke disdainfully of the quackish nature of his cures, and sought to discredit his gatherings as erotically charged and dangerous occasions.

At length, prompted by their complaints, the French authorities sought to outlaw Mesmer's activities. His disciples, seeking to overturn the ban and confident of his cures, prevailed upon the King to set up a commission of the Royal Academy to adjudicate the quarrel. A distinguished body it was, too, numbering the chemist Lavoisier, the astronomer Bailly, and the American

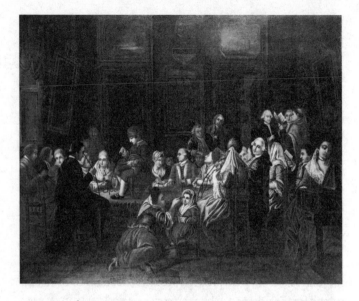

5. A group of patients mesmerized by Franz Anton Mesmer himself in Paris, 1778. (*Wellcome Library, London*)

ambassador to France, Benjamin Franklin, among its members. "Animal magnetism," they concluded, was a phantasm, a figment of Mesmer's and his patients' imagination, and his vaunted cures merely the product of credulity and suggestion. It was a verdict Mesmer bitterly resented, for he was every bit as convinced as other eighteenth-century theorists of hysteria and the nerves that he had identified a real physiological phenomenon, and that the magnetic force he mobilized was a genuine physical entity that worked by breaking up obstructions and reopening channels of communication in the recesses of the body.

Resent it he might, but Mesmer and mesmerism were now branded as a species of charlatanry. That hysteria might perhaps be a disorder of the mind rather than the brain and the nerves, that there might be value in treatments that operated at the level of the psyche, were thoughts neither he nor his critics were willing to entertain. In the aftermath of the commission's report, Mesmer felt compelled to leave Paris, retreating into social and professional obscurity. Yet, despite its official rejection, mesmerism lived on, and during Victorian times would enjoy a remarkable underground popularity among the well-to-do and the chattering classes, even while medical men dismissed it as a worthless anathema. Charles Dickens and Wilkie Collins were but two examples of those drawn to its rituals. But the mesmeric trance was a source of entertainment and mystery, only occasionally drawing the support of mainstream physicians, and those who ventured into its waters, like the London professor John Elliotson, were promptly ostracized and professionally ruined for their pains.

IV

⚭

REFLEXLY MAD

The famous French philosopher Michel Foucault first rose to prominence by asserting that a Great Confinement of the mad was one of the defining features of the eighteenth century. Like many of his oracular pronouncements, the claim was factually mistaken, but on this occasion he was only off by a century or so. All across Western Europe and North America, the first half of the nineteenth century witnessed what David Rothman has called "the discovery of the asylum."[1] Differences in national cultures and political and social structures meant that the pathways to the incarceration of the insane in what was held to be a therapeutic isolation varied considerably, but the new commitment to locking up the lunatic, most often at state expense, could be seen in France and Germany just as easily as in England or the United States.

Here was a transformation of social practices that at the outset was marked by an almost utopian optimism about what the new asylums could accomplish. Experiments with a variety of non-medical interventions collectively known as "moral treatment" led contemporaries to conclude that grave forms of mental illness were in reality more curable than the physical disorders with which the medical profession generally wrestled. In legislatures, in the popular press, and in the writings of medical men, it was Bedlam madness that drew most of the attention. The problems of the raving, delusional, hallucinating madman, and the withdrawn, desolate, perhaps suicidal melancholic, for a time largely displaced the hysteric from the public stage.

Nor did the asylum vanish from the scene as the Victorian age grew to maturity. On the contrary, what had often begun as a series of small, charismatically run therapeutic establishments morphed into a vast network of museums for the collection and exhibition of the ever expanding ranks of the irrational. Legions of lunatics emerged to populate the wards of what increasingly came to be seen as warehouses of the unwanted, and a whole new group of medical specialists—variously calling themselves asylum superintendents, medical psychologists, alienists, and eventually psychiatrists—emerged to minister to these diseased minds, and to rule like petty autocrats over the miniature kingdoms of the mad that now pock-marked the countryside.

Yet, even when professional and public attention was largely focused elsewhere, the nervous and the hysterical did not entirely disappear. On the contrary, nervous patients remained a staple of general practice in the early 1800s. In an overcrowded medical marketplace, demanding hysterics who sought attention for a wide range of mysterious and recalcitrant ailments could on purely economic grounds prove a boon, however frustrating their ailments might otherwise seem. Nervous irritability and strain provided an all-purpose explanation for the hysteric's troubles, one that comfortingly located her (or more occasionally his) complaints in a somatic framework that satisfied both doctor and patient. If such patients became overtly delusional or violent, or threatened self-harm, the general practitioner now had the option of referring them to his professional brethren who oversaw the madhouses. But, in the meantime, the doctor had at his disposal a variety of weapons to employ in the treatment of the sane but troubled hysterics who sought his attention—at least if they had the good fortune and good manners to come from the affluent classes.

There were pills, of course, all manner of pills. Nerve tonics. Iron. Strychnine. Quinine (or the Peruvian bark). Arsenic might be mobilized to provide a therapeutic jolt to shattered nerves. "Blue pills"—calomel, or mercurous chloride—might be employed to purge the nervous system of its toxins. (Benjamin Rush, the first American physician to write on diseases of the mind, was emphatic in his endorsement: "Mercury acts in this disease by abstracting morbid excitement from the brain to the mouth…conveys morbid action out of the body by the mouth, and thus restores the mind to its native seat in the brain."[2]) And then there were the opiates—laudanum, morphine, and the like—all of which possessed, as a contemporary guide for the laity put it, "the wonderful properties of mitigating pain, inducing sleep, allaying inordinate action, and diminishing morbid irritability."[3] There were pills to produce vomits. Diuretics. Aperients. And in the first half of the nineteenth century, until medical confidence in the remedy plummeted, there was bleeding, by lancet, cupping, or leeches.

Still other therapeutic possibilities beckoned: the bracing effects of tonics could be reinforced by a change of scene—sea air, perhaps, or the pure air of the Alps, combined with the distractions of new and pleasing surroundings. Cheyne's prescriptions of bathing and drinking the sulfurous waters at Bath were updated. German spas became a particular favorite of nervous patients and their professional advisers, but there emerged all manner of hydrotherapeutic establishments catering to the nervous in less exotic domestic settings as well. Water was, for many, a sovereign remedy, employed by medical men and lay speculators alike. It could be hot, cold, or tepid; sprayed, soaked in, or administered through wet sheets or towels; or even drunk for its mineral content. Nervous irritation could thus be calmed, and then the body given new vigor, perhaps by a cold bath or shower. Hydrotherapy was an all-purpose remedy, and its only drawbacks were its associations with quackery (something that deterred many mainstream physicians from employing it), and the fact that, whatever temporary relief it offered, ultimately most patients lost faith in its healing powers.

Yet hysterical patients, while often lucrative, seldom seemed to get better. As often as not they blamed their continued debility on the failures of those treating them, and sought out another opinion, sometimes consulting a dozen or more practitioners in turn. Such antics, and the implied reproach to medicine's powers, scarcely endeared them to the profession. And in other ways they were perceived to be singularly unrewarding patients: peevish, constantly complaining, with a mass of chronic, non-specific troubles, their protracted invalidism and frequent ingratitude were wearisome and provoking.

If patients could (and did) blame their doctors for their troubles, medical men could return the favor with interest. Discomfort over the impotence of their remedies against such intractable disorders could easily spill over into anger at those who seemed so determined to remain invalids, and more than a few doctors began to harbor the suspicion that their hysterical patients were perhaps not such innocent victims after all. What if hysteria was not a purely somatic disorder? What if it were a psychological condition, even a willful retreat into illness?

Then the very nature of the therapeutic encounter must and did change, for these men regarded the very notion of a psychological illness (in Szaszian fashion, *avant la lettre*) as a contradiction in terms, a category mistake. Either symptoms were the product of a real, physiologically based pathology, or they were a form of fakery, a manipulative malingering and deceit that deserved scorn and moral opprobrium, if not worse. And worse was indeed forthcoming, in the form of treatments whose sadistic qualities hint at the not very deeply buried professional fury that may have prompted them. Take, for example, W. Tyler Smith's prescriptions for the nervous, menopausal women who crowded his waiting room and consultation chambers. Their erotic and nervous symptoms ought to be dealt with, he suggested, "by a course of injections of ice water into the rectum, introduction of ice into the vagina, and leeching of the labia and cervix." His approving comments on the latter intervention rather give the game away: "The suddenness with which leeches applied to this part fill themselves considerably increases the good effect of their application, and for some hours after their removal, there is an oozing of blood from the leech bites."[4]

At about the same time, Robert Brudenell Carter set up shop as a young general practitioner in the then leafy environs of Leytonstone, east of London. In later years Brudenell Carter would go on to achieve distinction as an ophthalmologist, but, like many an impecunious newly minted doctor, in his twenties he had perforce to take whatever customers presented themselves. As for many of his fellow practitioners, these included a not inconsiderable number of cases of hysteria. As his frustrations with these patients (who were almost all women) mounted, he came to change his views on what was wrong with them, and finally ventured to put his ideas and conclusions into print.[5]

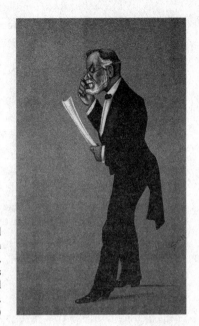

6. Robert Brudenell
Carter (1828–1918) as an
ophthalmologist and an old man,
many years removed from his
youthful book on hysteria and
its treatment. (*Wellcome Library,
London*)

The impact of one's emotional state on one's bodily health
had been a cliché of Hippocratic and Galenic medicine. Strong
emotions could disrupt the equilibrium of the body, as could
readily be seen in cases of extreme fright or fear, and Brudenell
Carter suggested that they could likewise produce the "primary paroxysm" that marked the onset of hysteria. Here was
the important source of the far greater frequency of hysteria
among the female of the species. For "the general predominance of reasoning and feeling [among men and women]
respectively, is universally acknowledged."[6] Men think, women
feel. And yet civilization insisted that women, "if unmarried
and chaste," must suppress the most powerful emotion of all,
"sexual desire." While

man has such facilities for its gratification, that as a source of disease it is almost inert against him, ladies labour under the modern necessity for its entire concealment...[Thus] it is likely to produce hysteria in a larger number of the women subject to its influence than it would do if the state of society permitted its free expression.[7]

In and of itself, Brudenell Carter's conclusion that "the sexual emotions are those most concerned in the production of the disease"[8] did not necessitate a break with the idea that, at bottom, hysteria was a disorder rooted in the body. But he now introduced a distinction that made hysteria's ontological status much more suspect. The initial hysterical fit might indeed be traced back to physiology, but, as the natural history of the disorder unfolded, it underwent a subtle shift. By degrees, the primary disturbance developed secondary and then tertiary manifestations. Secondary attacks were provoked by the recall of the emotions that had produced the original attack, and could sometimes be deliberately induced by the patient. Tertiary attacks always took this form, being deliberately instigated by the patient:

Attacks of this kind may be distinguished from primary hysteria by the frequency with which they occur in the absence of any exciting cause; by their never being produced under circumstances which would expose the patient to serious discomfort or real danger, but at a time and place discreetly chosen for the purpose; and by observing the many little arrangements contrived in order to add to their effect...their number and variety depending upon the ingenuity of the performer, and the extent of her resources.[9]

These hysterical patients were thus simulating illness, often adopting into their performance symptoms inadvertently suggested by their medical attendant or by illnesses they had witnessed in other people. Such behaviors were deeply ingrained in the patients' psyches, and extraordinarily difficult to dislodge. The infliction of physical pain as a deterrent was useless, "since the patient herself often inflicts upon herself much more pain than any medical attendant could possibly propose."[10] But, for all that, tertiary hysteria was the product of "selfishness and deceptivity."[11] Indeed, such was the moral depravity of those exhibiting these symptoms that they arranged to satisfy their "prurient desires" by exploiting medical men's belief in the gynecological origins of their sufferings:

> I have … seen young unmarried women, of the middle class of society, reduced by the constant use of the speculum, to the mental and moral condition of prostitutes; seeking to give themselves the same indulgence by the practice of solitary vice; and asking every medical practitioner … to institute an examination of the sexual organs.[12]

Paragons of moral obliquity, most hysterical women were thus blameworthy, not sick. They were actresses, not real invalids, and yet they clung to their symptoms with a fierceness and persistence that defied and defeated most medical men's efforts to cure them. Brudenell Carter's repugnance in the face of what he clearly saw as "falsehoods" and manipulative malingering by those with "deadened moral sensibility" was palpable, and reflected a frustration that others who encountered such creatures also voiced. His anger manifested itself transparently in his therapeutic recommendations. The medical man had to maneuver to wear out "the moral endurance of the patient."[13] Neither sympathy nor alarm should be expressed, no matter how extreme the symptoms. Rather, he should "commence by a positive assertion that she has nothing at all the matter with her, and is, in reality, in perfectly good health; her ailments being, one and all, fraudulent imitations of real disease."[14] Against this deception, the doctor must wage "mental warfare," employing "humiliation and shame" and "threats of exposure" to encourage reformation. His must be a full frontal assault, admitting of no doubt or hesitation. "In all cases it will be necessary to use plain words, and to convey the idea of selfishness and falsehood by their simplest names, and not under the disguise of any polite and elegant periphrasis."[15] Anger or tears, indignation and violent resistance, must all be ignored, met with a calm authority that insists that it will be obeyed, and on no account should any concession be made to the "pretended illness."

The battle could be fierce and prolonged. It was best fought away from the comforts of the domestic hearth, where family members might succumb to the wily woman's manipulation of the symptoms of sickness, and, with misplaced sympathy, forestall the necessary firmness. Removal to the doctor's house was a sensible means of ensuring that no misguided sentiment could interfere. Victory would in the end go to the side that exhibited the most determination and fortitude. Precautions had to be taken against the "fatal error of neglecting real disease"[16]—and it was this requirement, at the last, that justified medical men undertaking the battle against a disorder that was not a real physical illness, and thus did not appear to belong in the medical arena. Members of all other professions were at risk of being deceived by fits, or episodes of bleeding, paralyses and pains, and thus of giving legitimacy and new life to symptoms that must at all costs be ignored and repressed. "The process," Brudenell Carter confessed, "is always troublesome, and often difficult, but I have yet to hear of the case, in which it would ultimately fail of success; and I offer it to my brethren as a remedy, which is, humanly speaking, certain, against one of the most unmanageable diseases they are ever called upon to contend with."[17]

It was a perspective on hysteria, Brudenell Carter acknowledged, that not just patients, but also their families, refused to countenance. The simulation of sickness was so convincing, the obduracy of the patients so difficult to break down, the conviction of the relatives that the young woman was of too elevated a moral standing to engage in such deceptions, that he could but seldom put his plans into practice. Moreover, like any other doctor, were he to take more than one "nervous" patient into his home at a time, he risked running afoul of the lunacy laws, which, in an effort to protect patients from abuse, now required that only licensed and inspected asylums could confine the insane. Soon enough, Brudenell Carter moved on, applying his medical talents to other, less trying, and more rewarding disorders.

If Brudenell Carter and other general practitioners who grew tired of wrestling with the recalcitrance of the hysterical patient were tempted to dismiss hysteria from the ranks of authentic illness, others were not so certain. Researches on the nature of the nervous system had gathered pace in the early decades of the nineteenth century, and new understandings of nervous function provided an alternative basis for accounting for hysteria, one that revived its classical connections to the womb and the female reproductive organs, and did so in a fashion that reinforced the notion that hysteria was necessarily a predominantly, almost exclusively, female complaint. Most emphatically, too, hysteria was a physiologically based (and thus genuine) illness.

To be sure, nineteenth-century medical men did not require the specialized neurological work of a Charles Bell, a Marshall

Hall, a Thomas Laycock, or a Johannes Müller to conclude that women were different, inferior specimens of humanity, a weaker sex whose inferiority was rooted firmly in their reproductive biology. For Victorian physicians, few facts were more incontestably established than that the female of the species was, as Carroll Smith-Rosenberg and Charles Rosenberg have felicitously put it, "the product and prisoner of her reproductive system."[18] Woman's place in society—her capacities, her roles, her behavior—was ineluctably linked to and controlled by the existence and functions of her uterus and ovaries. To the crises and periodicities of her reproductive organs could be traced all the peculiarities of her nature: the predominance of the emotional over the rational; her capacity for affection and aptitude for child-rearing; her preference for the domestic sphere; and her "natural" purity and moral sensibility. The instability of women's bodies that inescapably dogged their daily existence in turn profoundly affected female health, and formed the physiological foundation of her greater delicacy and fragility.

What the new work on the nerves contributed to the "scientific" demonstration of female difference and inferiority was a new way of conceptualizing and accounting for women's heightened emotional lability and vulnerability. The English mad-doctor, George Man Burrows, had claimed in 1828 that science had authoritatively demonstrated that "the functions of the brain are so intimately connected with the uterine system, that the interruption of any one process which the latter has to perform in the human economy may implicate the former."[19] At the time they were first written, such assertions rested upon little more than bluster. Subsequent experimental work on the nervous system, however, led to the development of the notion of "reflex action," and the associated notion of reflex irritability provided a novel way to account for women's heightened susceptibility to emotional disorder and mental disease. Puberty, pregnancy, parturition, lactation, menstruation, and the menopause—each added to the constant shock and strain on the female bodily system, prompting in all too many cases the shipwreck of the intellect, the collapse of the will, and the dissolution of all semblance of self-control. Hence women's susceptibility, in the words of the Harvard physician Horatio Storer, to a variety of mental defects of a hysterical sort with "neither homologue or analogue in man."[20] In general, "volition, voluntary motion and judgment were believed to be functions of the central nervous system [while] the bodily functions, including reproduction, were thought to be regulated by the reflex nervous system."[21] Women, who possessed a large and complicated reproductive apparatus and only small brains, were thus far more susceptible than the male of the species to the predominance of reflex action over rational thought.

From puberty onwards, the maturation of a woman's body produced a major alteration in her reproductive organs, which were intimately linked to her nervous system and thence to her brain. Henceforth, she was "obedient to a special law...the victim of periodicity, her life is one perpetual change." Latent "emotions, desires, and passions...are now established" and trouble looms. For the passions dependent upon these physical changes lurk "like the smoldering fires of the volcano, ready to burst forth at any exciting moment."[22] "Excitement" or disorders of the reproductive system thus imposed immense strain on the brain and nerves and could prompt hysteria or even outright insanity. "Just as we have special diseases of the pelvic organs in the female, so we may have functional diseases of the brain, of many and deceptive types, excited in her thereby."[23] Sex, whether coitus or masturbation, or even "improper excitement of the imagination," creates "nervous excitement and vascular turgescence of the uterine organs," which in turn "determine the character of the mental disorder, elevating certain of the moral sentiments, or of the intellectual manifestations to a state of extravagance." Hence "hysterical females."[24]

One particular group of medical men seized upon these ideas with relish, for such notions promised a considerable expansion of their role in ministering to the needs of their patients. For centuries, Western medicine had denigrated the very concept of specialization. Specialization was for "quacks," irregulars who battened upon public credulity and sold patent remedies for unmentionable venereal complaints, for diseases of the eye, or diabetes, or gout. (Specialists, of course, by laying claim to superior expertise, were a major competitive threat in an overcrowded medical marketplace in which the individual practitioner had a hard time standing out.) The rise of asylum medicine had represented one minor exception to this traditional view. Mad-doctors, though, were viewed with almost as much suspicion by their medical brethren as by the public at large, their motives and competence both seen as suspect. The primary weapon they employed against insanity—moral treatment—had been developed largely by laymen who saw little value in conventional medical therapeutics, and its focus on the social psychological manipulation of the patient's environment left scant space for treatments directed at the body. Alienists' distinctive practice as asylum-based doctors, with its heavily stigmatized and physically isolated patient population, was thus easily seen as atypical, and their specialism accordingly as being of little concern to the medical profession at large.

The suspicion that extended to other forms of specialism was rooted in part in crassly economic considerations. In the early nineteenth century, the individual doctor had a hard time standing out from the crowd. The fear of being labeled as following a trade had led medical practitioners to reinforce earlier prohibitions against advertising their wares, conduct seen as unseemly among men aspiring to gentlemanly status. Setting up as a specialist potentially offered a legitimate way of attracting patients, as long as the self-proclaimed expert could persuade prospective customers that he possessed more experience and skill than the general practitioner in ministering to particular forms of disease and debility. It was a strategy most readily pursued by those with an easily demarcated mode of practice, and among the first to seize the opportunity this situation presented were surgeon-accoucheurs.

Gynecologists, as they began to call themselves by the middle decades of the nineteenth century, posed a particularly potent threat to the general practitioner. They ministered, of course, to some of women's most intimate needs, and their presence at the delivery of children ensured them a recurring, highly visible, and crucial role in their patients' lives. The advance of gynecology as a medical specialty simultaneously produced and was dependent upon the increasing place of technology in the birth process, and in approaches to the diseases of women's reproductive organs. At a period in which the bankruptcy of traditional heroic therapeutics was becoming increasingly visible, prompting many physicians to embrace therapeutic nihilism and many patients to desert allopathic medicine for homeopathy, Thomsonianism, and a variety of other sectarian competitors, it was on advances in surgical technique and practice that orthodox medicine's continued hold on the public perhaps most crucially rested. In gynecology, as in surgery more generally, these advances derived, in the last analysis, from two crucial developments: the use of anesthesia, beginning in the 1840s; and the acceptance in the last third of the century (though not without a struggle) of Lister's emphasis on anti-sepsis. Anesthesia and anti-sepsis, particularly in combination, made the routine employment of invasive surgery possible for the first time, and allowed refinements of skills and capacities that constituted spectacular confirmation of medicine's claims to scientific legitimacy.

Among the gynecological operators of the 1850s, few were more enthusiastic and audacious than Isaac Baker Brown, whose technical skills (and willingness to risk his patients' lives) soon placed him in the forefront of the London medical elite. He was elected a fellow of the Royal College of Surgeons in 1848, and his operating theater soon became, in the admiring words of Thomas Wakley, editor of *the Lancet*, "one of the most attractive to the professional visitor in all London—admiration being invariably evoked by his brilliant dexterity and the power he displayed in the use of his left hand when operating on the female perineum."[25] The publication of *Surgical Diseases of Women* in 1854, and his major role in the foundation of St Mary's Hospital, marked further steps on his path to professional prominence, culminating in his election, in 1865, as President of the Medical Society of London.

In the early 1850s, Baker Brown became one of the first to use chloroform in midwifery and in obstetrical operations. He pioneered new techniques for repairing vaginal and rectal fistulae, and for dealing with the prolapsed uterus. And, notwithstanding the deaths of his first three patients, he experimented enthusiastically with ovariotomy as a cure for "ovarian dropsy."

The predictable result of what the editor of the *Lancet* termed "his celebrity as an operator at once bold, ingenious, and successful"[26] was to bring him a steady influx of affluent and aristocratic patients, so that by 1858 he felt secure enough to withdraw from his association with St Mary's and to establish his own proprietary hospital, The London Home for Surgical Diseases of Women.

Like many of his colleagues engaged in the treatment of the female genitals, Baker Brown had been repeatedly frustrated and foiled in those cases in which physical pathology was complicated "with hysterical and other nervous affections..." Such women, he said, echoing some of Brudenell Carter's complaints, "defied my most carefully conceived efforts at relief."[27] His sense of frustration was relieved, however, when he read Brown-Sequard's lectures on "The Physiology and Pathology of the Central Nervous System," published in the *Lancet* the same year the London Home opened its doors. For the first time a line of attack on these recalcitrant cases occurred to him. In keeping with the contemporary doctrine of reflex irritability, the French physiologist had argued that damage to the central nervous system might be caused by over-excitement of the peripheral nerves. Baker Brown immediately saw the relevance to his own practice: the source of his patients' hysteria and nervous complaints must surely lie in a pernicious and all-but-unmentionable habit, "peripheral excitement of the pudic nerve"—or, to put it bluntly, female masturbation.

In invoking masturbation as a cause of hysteria and other forms of insanity, Baker Brown was scarcely advancing a novel hypothesis. Masturbatory insanity had been a staple of early nineteenth-century psychiatric texts, and had acquired new credibility in many quarters through the growing emphasis on the importance of the conservation of energy. In other hands, this theory had already been invoked to justify a number of painful, or more accurately sadistic, "remedies." Particularly popular was the "continual application of the strongest caustics to the seat of the irritation,"[28] in an effort to dissuade the patient from the filthy habit. Characteristically, however, Baker Brown scorned these sorts of half measures as wholly inadequate to "destroy such deep-seated nerve irritation" and proceeded at once to "a surgical test, by removing the cause of excitement," the woman's clitoris.[29]

This desperate remedy was justified, in Baker Brown's eyes, by the danger that nervous exhaustion posed to the whole system. Loss of nerve power as a result of masturbation was, he assured his readers, followed successively by "hysteria, spinal irritation, hysterical epilepsy, cataleptic fits, epileptic fits, idiotcy [sic], mania, and finally death." And the record of his operative results between 1858 and 1866 proved that "the treatment must be the same whether we wish to cure functional disturbance, arrest organic disease, or, finally, if we have only a chance of averting death itself."[30] Patients deemed suitable cases for treatment were operated upon immediately; he paused only to ensure that they had "been placed completely under the influence of chloroform" before "the clitoris is freely excised either by scissors or knife."[31] The results, according to Baker Brown himself, were enormously gratifying, and, within a month, "it is difficult for the uninformed, or nonmedical, to discover any trace of an operation."[32] Idiots, epileptics, hysterics, paralytics, the young and the old, all proved readily curable through surgical intervention. Even in cases of nymphomania, where "under medical treatment, of how short duration is…too frequently the benefit," success was all but guaranteed: indeed, "in no case am I so certain of a permanent cure…for I have never after my treatment seen a recurrence of the disease."[33]

Despite, or perhaps because of, these vaunted successes, and notwithstanding its apparent conformity with some of the central assumptions of mid-Victorian medical theory, Baker Brown's work brought him opprobrium rather than the hoped-for fame. Within a year of his book's appearance, both clitoridectomy and its author had been consigned to the outer darkness. Why was this?

Not, for all appearances, because of the cruelty or failures of the treatment. As Elaine Showalter points out in *The Female Malady*: "The mutilation, sedation, and psychological intimidation…seems to have been an efficient, if brutal, form of reprogramming…"[34] and, in any event, the issue of inefficacy was never seriously pursued in the storm of criticism Baker Brown's work raised. The treatment was certainly brutal, as is made clear in the description given by one of Baker Brown's former assistants:

> Two instruments were used: the pair of hooked forceps which Mr Brown always uses in clitoridectomy, and a cautery iron…The clitoris was seized by the forceps in the usual manner. The thin edge of the red hot iron was then passed around its base until the origin was severed from its attachments, being partly cut or sawn, and partly torn away. After the clitoris was removed, the nymphae on each side were severed in a similar way by a sawing motion of the hot iron. After the clitoris and nymphae were got rid of, the operation was brought to a close by taking the back of the iron and sawing the surfaces of the labia and the other parts of the vulva which had escaped the cautery, and the instrument was rubbed down backwards and forwards till the parts were more effectually destroyed than when Mr Brown uses the scissors to effect the same result.[35]

But the brutality of the surgery was likewise not the central issue, and scarcely could be, since some of Baker Brown's fiercest critics themselves used treatments that were every bit as unpleasant with their own female patients. Instead, it was the "ethics" of Baker Brown's behavior that drew down on his head the almost universal wrath of his colleagues. In fact, close attention to the record reveals that, even before the appearance of his book, Baker Brown's activities had drawn unfavorable comment from influential segments of the medical press. Mid-nineteenth-century medical practitioners could lay only a precarious claim to gentlemanly status, and medical elites were thus extraordinarily sensitive about behavior that threatened the profession's social standing. Baker Brown's activities raised this vital issue in multiple and mutually reinforcing ways.

He had aggressively and repeatedly sought public attention for and approval of his activities. In early 1866, for example, before his book on clitoridectomy appeared in print, he had arranged with a friendly reporter for the *Standard* for a hyperbolic article on "An Admirable Institute—The London Surgical Home." This immediately drew sharp criticism from the editor of the *British Medical Journal*, who commented tartly: "We doubt whether the profession will approve of the way in which this particular institution is brought before the public...A superfluous amount of self-laudation is not always a real recommendation."[36] Baker Brown failed to take the hint. A few issues later, the *British Medical Journal* returned to the attack: the recent annual report of the London Surgical Home was permeated by "a regrettable spirit of exaggeration..." And his new book on clitoridectomy, while demonstrating that "the operation may be of value in certain forms of nervous disease," made similarly wild and unsupported claims. Equally unforgivable was the presentation of subject matter fit only for the eyes of fellow medical men in a binding more suited "to a class of works which lie upon drawing room tables."[37] The impression that Baker Brown was seeking lay, rather than professional, approval was only accentuated by the appearance in the *Church Times* of an article endorsing his operation and urging clergymen to recommend it to their parishioners; and by the claim that Baker Brown had sent the annual report of the London Surgical Home "to half the nobility in the kingdom."[38] And, when Baker Brown again resorted to barely disguised advertising in the public press, planting another laudatory story touting his unique remedy in cases of insanity (on this occasion in *The Times* on December 15, 1866), the editors finally lost all patience, and referred his activities to the Commissioners in Lunacy.

Baker Brown thus proved fatally unwilling to abandon a line of conduct that deeply offended professional norms. His relentless pursuit of publicity smacked of the tradesman, an association that medical men (especially surgeons) were desperately anxious to live down. In the fiercely competitive medical world of mid-century London, advertising—direct or thinly disguised—threatened both the economic interests and the status of the profession. Accordingly, few behaviors were so predictably stigmatized and anathematized. At least equally serious was Baker Brown's preference for lay approval over the opinion of his professional peers. For this raised the specter of quackery, an association rendered the more plausible by the extraordinary array of hitherto untreatable conditions that Baker Brown claimed to cure.

By the close of 1866, the London medical elite was all but unanimously turning on someone who had, till recently, been one of its leading lights. As Michael Clark has rightly argued, the physician's moral and pastoral responsibilities were an essential—perhaps the essential—foundation of the Victorian medical man's claims to authority and prestige. Anything that cast even a shadow upon the appearance of moral rectitude and strict probity simultaneously threatened the profession's paramount concern with safeguarding the basis of its social standing and mandate. It was his violation of this "first principle of the physician's professional conduct"[39] that destroyed Baker Brown. For the injunction to uphold the basis of professional honor was always likely to be enforced with particular force and fury in the case of gynecology, a specialty whose practitioners, as the editor of the British Medical Journal put it, "beyond other [medical] men, are not only the guardians of life, but, by force of circumstance, often also the guardians of female honour and purity."[40]

The very precariousness of the position of the gynecologists, who had only just "emerged from the difficulties and clouds under which we lay during previous centuries," made it essential, in T. H. Tanner's words, that the Obstetrical Society should demonstrate to "the public that their health in our hands, as men of honour and gentlemen, is safe."[41] As men, and, more particularly, as medical men, gynecologists possessed extraordinary power over the weaker sex; yet their social mandate to exercise that power would rapidly evaporate were they to use their authority irresponsibly and "unethically." As Seymour Haden put it, in proposing the notion to expel Baker Brown from the Obstetrical Society:

> we have constituted ourselves, as it were, the guardians of [women's] interests, and in many cases...the custodians of their honour. We are, in fact, the stronger, and they the

weaker. They are obliged to believe all that we tell them. They are not in a position to dispute anything we say to them, and we therefore may be said to have them at our mercy... Under these circumstances, if we should depart from the strictest principles of honour, if we should cheat or victimize them in any shape or way, we would be unworthy of the profession of which we are members.[42]

Quite unambiguously, then, Baker Brown's conduct constituted "a breach of faith with every individual member of the profession...";[43] a betrayal of trust that, without a forceful response from the guardians of professional morality, might have delivered a body blow to the reputation for moral rectitude and probity upon which the profession's privileged place in the division of labor ultimately rested. Hence the harsh and unforgiving treatment by his peers. His would not prove to be the last occasion, however, when gynecologists sought to claim the treatment of hysteria as their own.

V

AMERICAN NERVOUSNESS

War, as the bumper sticker would have it, is not good for children and other living things. For medics, though, it is another matter entirely. The wounds of warfare, it goes without saying, require much medical attention—to keep up the morale of the troops, if not actually to cure many of those treated. (Prior to the spread of aseptic surgery, battlefield mortality was frightful, and medicine's weapons against infectious diseases, which regularly decimated the troops, were equally weak and unsatisfactory.) But beyond that, war allows army medics to observe the impact of all sorts of trauma on the human body, an array of naturalistic experiments from which much can potentially be learned, and which could never be replicated on a similar scale in normal times, even among such vulnerable populations as the mentally ill and the mentally retarded.

The American Civil War, one of the first modern, mechanized wars, and one that went on for years, producing massive quantities of dead and wounded, provides a classic illustration of this thesis. Prominent figures in military medicine seized on their experiences to learn new lessons about the pathology of living bodies, lessons they subsequently drew upon and exploited in the years following the war. The Philadelphia society doctor Silas Weir Mitchell, and his colleagues W.W. Keen and George Morehouse, produced a monograph on *Gunshot Wounds and Other Injuries of Nerves*, and, in the aftermath of the war, Mitchell set up shop as part of a new breed of medical specialists, neurologists, a branch of the healing arts in which he was soon joined by, among others, the man who had served as Surgeon General of the Union Army, William Alexander Hammond.

American neurology, as a clinical specialty, can thus trace its origins to the impact of war. That was true in another sense, of course, for many of the patients who thronged the waiting rooms of these new "nerve specialists" were soldiers who were casualties of the fighting. Some had obvious traumatic injuries to their heads, their spinal cords, or their peripheral nervous system. Others had wounds that were more difficult to trace, perhaps, as few dared to hint, even imaginary or the product of the psychological trauma they had experienced. But there was still another group of patients who began to show up in increasing numbers, and here there could be no question of battlefield trauma, physical or psychological—for these were members of the fairer sex, hysterics who descended on the new group of specialists as though they represented manna from Heaven. General practitioners had failed them. Gynecologists had not yet come up with a distinctive new therapy for their nervous clientele, though they would soon claim to have done so. If the neurologists were the new cutting edge of scientific medicine, if they knew more than anyone else about the disorders of the brain and the nerves, why then, who better to treat hysteria?

Willing or not, neurologists thus found themselves drawn into the maelstrom of functional nervous disorders, whether

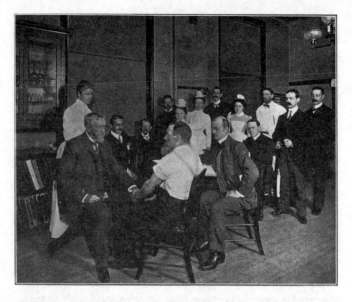

7. Silas Weir Mitchell (1829–1914), Philadelphia neurologist and novelist, the inventor of the "rest cure," who grew rich from the hysterics and neurasthenics who flocked to consult him. He is shown here examining a Civil War veteran at the Clinic of the Orthopedic Hospital of Philadelphia. (*Wellcome Library, London*)

among army veterans or among wealthy society matrons (and their adolescent daughters), all importuning a diagnosis for their disorder, and the most modern, up-to-date, scientific treatment. Perforce they had to respond, and, in any event, the nascent state of their specialism, with its associated economic vulnerabilities, meant that they could scarcely afford to turn away such lucrative and persistent patients.

On yet another front, neurologists' focus on disorders of the brain and the nervous system at least implicitly extended to a claim to expertise with respect to all forms of nervous and mental disease. In general, the problem of drawing clear distinctions between neurological and psychiatric disease was something Victorians wrestled with, but without making much progress. So, at least in theory, neurology was a rival to the asylum doctors, with their captive population of the insane. And, in practice, there can be little doubt that there was a fair degree of overlap between the patients who fetched up in neurological waiting rooms, and those who found themselves confined involuntarily in asylums. Certainly, the neurologists increasingly thought of themselves as embracing this whole spectrum of diseases, and conceived of themselves as infinitely better trained and more scientific than their professional counterparts—men they saw as detached from "scientific medicine," having chosen to lock themselves into the asylums they presided over almost as securely as the patients they confined. They were, sneered the New York neurologist Edward Spitzka, experts in heating systems, running asylum farms, and disposing of sewage, "experts at everything except the diagnosis, pathology, and treatment of insanity."[1] As neurologists gave voice to their perceived superior knowledge and skills in this fashion, they inevitably provoked growing antagonism with the alienists, the branch of the mad-doctoring trade that practiced in asylums.

By the 1870s, the two groups of specialists were openly sniping at one another, and the feud grew nastier yet in the following decade. Simultaneously, however, both found themselves fending off yet another group of medical men who trespassed onto this territory. For the ignominious end of Isaac Baker Brown had not driven all the hysterical patients from the gynecologists' waiting rooms, nor extinguished the interest of many of that specialty's membership in ministering to so numerous and lucrative a clientele. The claimed connection between womb, ovaries, and brain now prompted the invention of another surgical remedy for hysteria.

The new operation, "normal ovariotomy," was designed to produce an artificial menopause. Its originator, an American surgeon from Rome, Georgia, with the rather apt name of Battey, announced his breakthrough in 1873 in suitably apocalyptic tones: "I have felt it to be my duty to…carve [sic] out for myself a new pathway through consecrated ground…I have invaded the hidden recesses of the female organism and snatched from its appointed set a glandular body, whose mysterious and wonderful functions are of the highest interest to the human race."[2] Others, of course, had previously "snatched" ovaries from their appointed seat. Battey's originality consisted in deliberately extending the operation to the extirpation of *healthy* organs. Hence the term "normal" ovariotomy, a choice of language he later came to regret.

Although Battey offered his operation as an effective treatment for a variety of pathological conditions that were held to depend upon the periodicities that plagued menstruating women, its allegedly marvelous curative properties were soon concentrated upon the treatment and cure of nervous ailments. As an operation on the external genitalia, Baker Brown's clitoridectomy could be undertaken even in the pre-antisepsis era, with only occasionally fatal complications from fulminating infections. But ovariotomy—or, as it was also called, oophorectomy—became technically feasible on a major scale only once the importance of antisepsis had been grasped and generally accepted. Even then, during the first decade of the operation, mortality rates averaged one-third of all cases treated, so that those experimenting with the treatment found themselves generally condemned, and at times even ostracized.

By the 1880s, however, death rates had declined quite markedly, to what were regarded as more acceptable levels (Battey himself, for example, reported a series of 70 cases in 1886 with only 2 deaths and 68 "recoveries"), and, with the technical feasibility of the operation now established, a veritable mania for ovariotomy swept the United States and (to a lesser extent) Britain. The precise number of operations performed during the 1880s and 1890s can never be established, since they were, with a few exceptions, confined to private practice, or to general hospitals; but the English surgeon Lawson Tait himself performed several hundred, and, judging from the published cases alone, several thousand and quite possibly tens of thousands of women must have submitted themselves to the surgeon's knife.

Almost all of them were those who hovered on the borderlands of insanity, the inhabitants of what the British doctor Mortimer Granville referred to as "Mazeland, Dazeland, and Driftland."[3] For the most part, asylum superintendents simply blocked access to institutionalized patients, reluctant to allow competitors into an arena they sought to monopolize, and fearful of the backlash from the public at large were they to allow hazardous experimentation on their captive population. It was thus hysterics and those who, in the words of the eminent Philadelphia gynecologist William Goodell, "hovered on the narrow borderland that separates hysteria from insanity,"[4] who were the usual beneficiaries of Battey's operation, typically middle- and upper-class women. Doctor, patient, and family could agree, with few qualms, that, as a way station on the road to chronic insanity, hysteria called for drastic measures designed to secure what Goodell termed "a ray of hope," perhaps the "only chance," of staving off a life of permanent invalidism or, worse still, the stigma of confinement in an asylum.[5]

Once the operation became widely known, doctors reported that they were besieged by women begging for the treatment. Some of these statements may have been self-serving, a means of heading off criticism from the rest of the medical profession or from the public at large about the wisdom of persuading women to submit to such an irreversible operation, one that blighted forever the prospect that their patients could contribute to that most vital and sacred of feminine tasks, the propagation of the species. But it would be wrong to be too cynical. The reports came from so many quarters, from male and female physicians alike, that it is difficult to believe that they were simply invented. Besides, the spectacle of hysterics rushing to embrace a somatic account of their troubles is scarcely unknown in other times, even in our own. In this instance, the assault on the ovaries was in line with long-standing folk beliefs about the origins of women's emotional lability, beliefs that had acquired a new veneer of scientificity with the development of reflex theories of nervous action. And ovariotomies at the very least served to end the endless cycle of pregnancies and parturition that was the lot of many Victorian women, a secondary gain some of the patients may deliberately have sought.

Neurologists, who had long been harshly critical of asylum superintendents for being out of touch with the cutting edge of medical advances, were even more contemptuous of the claims of the advocates of sexual surgery. Wharton Sinkler, an eminent Philadelphia neurologist, commented sardonically:

> A first successful abdominal section seems to have the same effect upon an operator as the taste of blood upon the Indian tiger. A thirst insatiable is aroused, and life is spent in looking for new victims. Cases running into double and triple figures are cited, where all the worst features of the most stubborn

nature have disappeared, as though the surgeon's knife were gifted with the power of an enchanter's wand.[6]

Reasserting that insanity and related conditions were the product of "nerve exhaustion" or disease, and hence belonged securely within the neurologist's province, other neurologists accused their colleagues of having fallen into a trap: "We are liable to be misled by what we see," particularly in cases of hysteria, "which very much simulate organic disease."[7] But such cases merely counterfeited organic mischief, while the true causes of the disorder resided in the nervous system.

Consistent with these judgments, leading neurologists routinely denounced ovariotomy as a treatment for hysteria as simply a mutilation, a variety of "heroic surgery, of...the most flagrant and pernicious form," whose "evil and uselessness can not be too strongly condemned."[8] Others were a little more restrained, though scarcely less critical. The New York neurologist Archibald Church argued that, even were one to assume that the procedure had some therapeutic value, it was far too drastic and dangerous to be employed against "a comparatively hopeful malady [like hysteria]"; while his Boston colleague Robert Edes cautioned that, despite all the exaggerated claims, "the relief is either none at all or only such as may be temporarily obtained from any strong impression whose effect is hopefully awaited."[9]

By the mid-1890s, these doubts had spread among elite gynecologists, and, as a treatment for hysteria, ovariotomies rapidly declined in popularity. Accumulating experience was discrediting the earlier optimistic claims about the operation's therapeutic impact, and increased knowledge about the importance of "glandular secretions" to women's health cast doubt on the wisdom of extirpating the ovaries. At least as important were growing ethical qualms that arose, ironically, from these male doctors' beliefs about woman's place in society. The claim to be proceeding in the hysterical woman's best interests "was hard to square with the general belief that 'ovariotomy' ruins a woman in all the essentials of womanhood." For moral reasons, "a mutilated woman" could not hope to marry. Who would have her? Without the possibility of procreation, a woman who engaged in sexual relations was little better than a whore. The gynecologist who brought about this parade of horribles could thus count himself, in the words of Howard Kelly of Johns Hopkins, the leading gynecologist of his age, "the destroyer of everything that makes a woman's life worth living."[10]

While gynecologists continued to see and treat the hysterical, their new claims to possess a distinctive treatment for the disease were severely damaged by this episode. Neurologists, by contrast, confidently proclaimed that their specialty was developing an ever more elaborate understanding of the nervous system and its disorders, and that they had an impressive array of treatments for these conditions, all capable of stimulating and restoring nervous action. The nervous system was increasingly seen as mediated through electrical signals, and for a decade or two electrotherapy in its various forms became a distinctive feature of neurological practice. Shiny and impressive chrome and brass machines delivered jolts of static electricity, and faradic currents were likewise employed to shake up the system, rearranging, as the neurologists solemnly assured their patients, the molecular structure of their bodies and simultaneously affecting the reflex actions of the nervous system. Drugs, too—ergot, strychnine, chloral, the bromides, arsenic, caffeine, Indian hemp, the opiates, and various proprietary tonics—were touted for their alternative value in stimulating and calming the nerves.

And diet and regimen were mobilized in the cause. American neurologists bemoaned the trials of dealing with the hysterical and the nervous. Silas Weir Mitchell spoke of hysterics as a "hated charge" of his specialty, and lamented that "hysteria" might better be termed "mysteria."[11] But he agreed with his New York colleague George Beard that "nervousness is a physical not a mental state, and its phenomena do not come from emotional excess or excitability or from organic disease but from nervous debility and irritability."[12]

General practitioners, like much of the public at large, were in many cases not convinced. To be sure, hysterics and nervous invalids exhibited many signs of suffering. Their complaints were loud and long, and their apparent physical symptoms—nervous prostration, fits, headaches, paralyses, floods of tears, and exhibitions of emotional lability, insomnia, and invalidism—were dramatic and disturbing. But were they real or imaginary? To be sure, they were tenaciously held on to, often at considerable cost. But these querulous creatures visibly enjoyed all sorts of secondary gains alongside these primary losses. Complaints that hysterical women were deceitful, manipulative, selfish creatures permeated many medical discussions of the problem they represented, one reason the British physician F. C. Skey recommended that they be treated with "fear and the threat of personal chastisement."[13] Their tricks and tantrums were, in the words of the leading English alienist of the period Henry Maudsley, a form of "moral perversion," and their resort to the sick bed a sham, "when all the while their only paralysis is a paralysis of the will."[14] Were these hysterical women in reality cynical malingerers, whose troubles were all "in their minds"?

It was a charge Weir Mitchell and his neurological colleagues fiercely resisted, and the more they insisted, drawing upon their prestige as those with the most expertise in the study of the nerves, that hysteria and allied complaints were genuine disorders of the body, the more the neurotic flocked to their consulting rooms. By way of consolation, hysteria was undoubtedly more treatable than the scleroses, the paralyses, the tics and epileptic fits, and the depressing array of tertiary syphilitics that were otherwise the neurologists' lot. And the legitimacy the "nerve doctors" conferred on the disorder ensured an ever large pool of patients, most from highly affluent and thus ultra-desirable circles. Mitchell's patients, for example, besides an array of society's *grandes dames*, included such prominent figures as Jane Addams, Winifred Howells, Edith Wharton, and Charlotte Perkins Gilman, and his ministrations to their needs made him an extremely wealthy man. Gilman skewered him and his rest cure in her novella, *The Yellow Wallpaper*, written in 1890 and published two years later. As she wrote in her journal, the enforced inactivity and complete absence of mental stimulation that Weir Mitchell enforced brought her "so near the borderline of mental ruin that I could see over." (Gilman sent her "fiction" to her doctor, who never acknowledged receiving it.)

By no means all the "nervous" patients who fetched up in the American neurologists' consulting rooms were women. For a brief period, the nervous man posed something of a challenge, for the nerve doctors were reluctant to extend the label of hysteria to encompass the male of the species, and the eighteenth-century male analogue, hypochondria, had by now acquired much of its modern meaning, an obsession with imaginary ills. Mitchell's New York colleague George Beard soon provided an intellectual solution to the difficulty. Nervous men, he announced, were suffering from neurasthenia—literally,

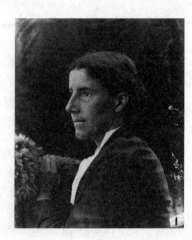

8. Charlotte Perkins Gilman (1860–1935), one of Silas Weir Mitchell's best-known patients. (*Schlesinger Library, Radcliffe Institute, Harvard University*)

weakness of the nerves—a condition brought on by overwork and overstress.

A century and a half earlier, George Cheyne had spoken of "the English malady," and had made what foreigners had considered a reproach—the heightened susceptibility of the English to hysterical disorders—a marker of England's prosperity, success, civilization, and refinement. Beard now spoke of "American nervousness" in analogous terms, as a maker of national superiority. American women, he noted complacently, were far and away the most beautiful in the world, their faces exhibiting an unparalleled combination of "delicacy, fineness, and mobility of expression."[15] Where "the English face is molded, the American is chiseled ... the superior fineness and delicacy of organization of the American woman ... revealing itself in the play of the eyes, the voice, in the response of the facial muscles, in gait, and dress, and gesture," but also in heightened susceptibility to nervous prostration.[16] Among Americans, male and female alike, it was the country's economic and cultural superiority that provoked so many nervous crises. The constant striving for success; the speed of modern life as exemplified by the telegraph and the steam engine; the excitement induced by the periodical press; the hurry of social change as unfettered capitalism allied to the powers of science revolutionized production and all aspects of daily life; and the increased mental activity of women: these were unique features of nineteenth-century civilization, but features that were felt with their full force only in America. "American nervousness, like American invention or agriculture, is at once peculiar and pre-eminent."[17] Striving and succeeding, the entrepreneurial American was always at fever pitch. But human beings possessed a finite store of nervous energy. Those who overtaxed their systems ran down their batteries, overloaded their circuits, overdrew their accounts, bankrupted their nervous systems, and were prone to breakdown.

The source of these analogies is plain, as is their appeal. Neurasthenia was a disease of the distinguished, of the best and the brightest, of the wealthy and the cultured, for it was these segments of society who were most exposed to the stresses and pressures of modernity, whose nervous systems were stretched tightest, eventually to breaking point. Bankers, lawyers, doctors, titans of industry and commerce, those who worked with their brains, not their hands ("the civilized, refined, and educated," in Beard's apt summary, "not the barbarous and low-born and untrained"[18])—these were the gentlemen at greatest risk, and their nervous prostration was thus a sign of their superior endowments and attainments—a diagnosis and an etiology that flattered the neurasthenic while reassuring them that theirs was emphatically a real physical illness, not some sign of weak will or self-indulgence. He counted himself among its victims, and a distinguished list it was: William and Henry James, Louis Agassiz, Theodore Dreiser, and W. E. B. Du Bois among Americans; John Ruskin, Francis Galton, Joseph Lister, Arnold Toynbee, and John Bright in England, to cite only a handful of eminent men who suffered from grave "nervous prostration."

The symptoms of neurasthenia or nervous collapse were many and varied and little different, if at all, from the protean symptoms that marked its twin, hysteria: sleeplessness, indigestion, weakness of the eyes, uterine irritation, chronic indecisiveness, permanent anxiety, irrational fears, impotence, heaviness of loin and limb, headache, neuralgia, flushing and fidgetiness, spasms and paralyses, claustrophobia and fears of contamination, to name but a few. Their protean character was a reflection of the overuse or abuse of the brain, the stomach, and the reproductive system. The consequence was an irritation or exhaustion of the nerve force, which, via reflex action, produced neurasthenia's many and varied physical manifestations, a puzzling array of troubles that had yielded their secret underlying unity only to the neurologist's probing gaze.

It would be too simple to dub neurasthenia the male version of hysteria, not least because many women soon populated the ranks of the neurasthenic, just as not inconsiderable numbers of men continued to be diagnosed as cases of hysteria. If it is clear that there was some gender preference in the allocation of diagnostic categories, it is equally plain that no clear dividing lines could be drawn between the two. Hysteria and neurasthenia were both perceived as protean nervous complaints, and it was simply not possible then (just as it is impossible today) to draw any hard and fast boundary between the two. Both male and female "nervous invalids" flocked to the nerve doctors' waiting rooms, and patronized the growing number of hydropathic establishments and sanatoriums that emerged to provide extended periods of respite for the affluent and the idle who had succumbed to the pressures of civilized existence. Though the female hysteric occupied a more prominent place in literary and popular culture, "it is utterly erroneous," as Janet Oppenheim rightly reminds us, "to assume that Victorian doctors perceived the male half of the human race as paragons of health and vigor, while assigning all forms of weakness to women. They could not have done so, even had they wanted to, for the evidence exposing male nervous vulnerability was too familiar to the Victorian public for pretense."[19]

If hysteria and neurasthenia had the origins in a malnourished and overburdened nervous system, one that was often made manifest to the trained clinical eye in the form of a thin, tense, scrawny physique, the obvious solution was to build up the body in hopes of restoring the nerves. Hence the resort to tonics, and to efforts to build up the system. The basic problem was signified by the title of one of Weir Mitchell's best-selling guides to laymen about nervous disorders: *Wear and Tear, or Hints for the Overworked*. And their therapeutics was neatly encapsulated in another of his medical advice books, *Fat and Blood: An Essay on the Treatment of Certain Forms of Neurasthenia and Hysteria*. Both passed through multiple editions, disseminating the neurologists' message to a wide and eager audience.

Americans, Mitchell warned, were at risk of "overtaxing and misusing the organs of thought," a problem compounded by the sedentary existence that brain work implied. When the ill-used brain at length rebelled, hysteria and neurasthenia were the inevitable result. Young girls were particularly at risk, for mental resources that ought to be conserved and directed towards their vital role as future wives and mothers were being frittered away in misguided mental pursuits and excitements. The facts of physiology implied that "it were better not to educate girls at all between the ages of fourteen to eighteen, unless it can be done with careful reference to their bodily health."[20] Externally, the outcome of neglecting this scientific imperative was an unfortunate "hardness of line in form and feature"[21] mistakenly viewed as beautiful. More ominously, though, for the future of the American race, the outcome was nervous creatures whose "destiny is the shawl and the sofa, neuralgia, weak backs, and the varied forms of hysteria—that domestic demon which has produced untold discomfort in many a household." "Only the doctor knows," Mitchell continued, "what one of these self-made invalids can do to make a household wretched... [Hence] the woman who wears out and destroys generations of nursing relatives, and who, as Wendell Holmes has said, is like a vampire, slowly sucking the blood of every healthy, helpful creature within reach of her demands."[22]

Mitchell's views here reveal his own underlying hostility towards his hysterical patients, an attitude that was broadly shared among the "nerve doctors," but they are also revelatory of some of the secondary gains the hysterical woman might obtain from her symptoms, the shift in the balance of power in the home that illness could license and produce. Misogynistic as Mitchell's pronouncements may seem to the contemporary reader, they were typical of "informed" medical opinion on both sides of the Atlantic. Henry Maudsley, who ministered to a similarly elite clientele of nervous patients in late-nineteenth-century Britain, was equally outspoken about the dangers of higher education for women. Emphasizing once more that "the energy of the human body [was] a definite and not inexhaustible quantity," he warned that females

99

on the brink of womanhood could "not bear, without injury, an excessive mental drain as well as the natural physical drain which is so great at that time."[23] Should they seek to do so, the result could only be a multiplication of the number of hysterics and the creation of "a race of sexless beings [who would] carry on the intellectual work of the world, not otherwise than as sexless ants do the work and fighting of the community."[24] Presumably, Maudsley and Mitchell did not anticipate the emergence of a class of female warriors. But they were united in their conviction, as Maudsley put it, that women "cannot rebel successfully against the tyranny of their organization"; they cannot escape the fact that a woman "labours under an inferiority of constitution by a dispensation which there is no gainsaying ... This is not the expression of prejudice nor of false sentiment; it is a plain statement of a physiological fact."[25]

To be sure, Maudsley and Mitchell, and their fellow specialists, had male as well as female patients, and here, too, wear and tear on the nervous system could produce "disastrous" results. "Neural exhaustion" was particularly likely in early adulthood, and again in middle age, where, at the height of a man's powers, he might find his brain unexpectedly rebelling, refusing more overwork, and launching him into a career as a hysterical or nervous invalid. Irregular meals, lack of sleep, an excess of blood in the brain, the lack of physical exercise, these and other excesses could sprain the brain. Thus, those "unable or unwilling to pause in the career of dollar getting ... making haste to be rich," were all-too-likely to find themselves "wrecked and made unproductive for years or forever."[26]

For male and female alike (though in practice women disproportionately received the treatment), Mitchell prescribed a

remedy that followed directly from his diagnosis of the problem. Wear and tear needed repair by building up fat and blood,
and that desirable goal could most readily be attained by an
extended period of rest and force-feeding. Soon dubbed the "rest
cure," Mitchell's approach was rapidly adopted as the standard
approach to the hysterical and the neurasthenic on both sides
of the Atlantic. By its very nature, rest was something only the
affluent could afford—not seemingly a problem so long as
etiological theories located hysteria and its analogues predominantly among members of the upper classes (though, in reality,
hysteria and neurasthenia were surfacing increasingly among
the lower orders, a situation neither theory nor therapy made it
easy to acknowledge).

"Rest" meant something quite complex in this context.
Patients were to be sequestered away from their families, lest
well-meaning relatives interfered with what followed. Patients
were then confined to bed continuously for weeks at a time,
and fed almost continuously with vast quantities of fattening
foods. All reading and writing, and other forms of intellectual
stimulation, were banned. In place of exercise, patients received
massages or electrical treatments to stimulate their muscles and
hasten defecation (the better to permit renewed feeding). In the
beginning, when "the most absolute rest is desirable, I arrange
to have the bowels and water passed while lying down, and the
patient is lifted on to a lounge for an hour in the morning and
again at bedtime [sic], and then lifted back again into the newly
made bed."[27] The inactivity and high-calorie diets often resulted
in massive weight gain, something the nerve doctors viewed
as a thoroughly satisfactory outcome. Above all, the patient's
will was subject to the imperious commands of her medical
attendant—"her" because, as Mitchell himself noted, "for some

reason, the ennui of rest and seclusion is far better borne by women than by the other sex." [28]

"Rest," then, "is not at all their notion of rest. To lie abed half the day, and sew a little, and read a little, and be interesting as invalids and excite sympathy, is all very well, but when they are bidden to stay in bed a month, and neither to read, write, nor sew, and to have one nurse,—who is not a relative—then repose becomes…a somewhat bitter medicine"[29]—one that even the more compliant sex found hard to swallow. But one that worked. The rest cure was, all agreed, the most comprehensive "regular, systematic, and thorough attack" on the problems of hysteria and neurasthenia, especially when those disorders were complicated by a refusal to eat. Physicians all across America, Britain, and continental Europe hurried to embrace its principles.

Sir William Gull, a leading society physician in London had begun to draw attention to emaciated hysterical women as early as 1868, terming their disorder "hysteric apepsia." An 1873 paper of his relabeled the condition. He now termed it "Anorexia Nervosa (Apepsia Hysterica, Anorexia Hysterica)"[30] and it was the first of these terms that caught on. Not surprisingly, Gull was an enthusiast for the rest cure, as were colleagues such as William Playfair, Thomas Clifford Allbutt, and the wonderfully named Thomas Stretch Dowse. When Virginia Woolf had her first breakdown in 1904, her physician, Sir George Savage, subjected her to a mild version of the cure, an experience Woolf, like the American writer Charlotte Perkins Gilman (a patient of Mitchell's), found intolerable. The enforced infantilization, the absence of all intellectual nourishment or stimulation, the utter boredom, the attempts to suppress their own individuality were a source of horror and wretchedness, vividly represented in Gilman's short story "The Yellow Wallpaper," a literary document that ensured that Weir Mitchell's name would reverberate in feminist circles in our own century as the epitome of the brusque, misogynist, paternalistic Victorian nerve doctor. How most who underwent the treatment felt we cannot know, though, alongside the protestors, other women certainly pronounced themselves grateful for the ministrations of Mitchell and his colleagues, and felt improved or cured by the experience. Was this false consciousness, or perhaps just a demonstration that women, like men, are in substantial measure creatures and prisoners of their culture's assumptions and prescribed roles?

VI

⸎

A HYSTERICAL CIRCUS

I t was Jean-Martin Charcot (1825–93), the august Professor of Pathological Anatomy and later of Diseases of the Nervous System of the Paris Medical Faculty, the leading international neurologist of the nineteenth century, who made hysteria a spectacle and a circus. It was a scandalous circus that attracted the attention of *tout Paris*, one that regularly featured scantily clad women disporting themselves in unmistakably erotic cataleptic poses, or writhing and moaning in ways that mimicked orgasms on a public stage, before an understandably rapt audience—an audience soon drawn not just from the highest ranks of French society, but also from those attracted to Paris by news of these extraordinary *Leçons du Mardi*. The photographs of these occasions, captured in carefully staged arrangements before the supposedly objective lens of the camera and thus transmuted into indelible visual representations for a vastly greater virtual audience, have survived for later generations to inspect, and have become the iconic images of a disorder seen as at once sexual and feminine.

Yet Charcot thought of himself, and was acknowledged by his contemporaries, to be no nineteenth-century Mesmer, no marginal charlatan catering to depraved appetites (among patients and audience alike), but on the contrary a sober scientist, a man of genius, one of the leading contributors to the newly emerging science of the brain. His accomplishments first in internal medicine and then as a neurologist were legion, and had brought him czars and princes, great merchants and bankers, as his clients, in the process making him a very rich man. And, while his most famous hysterical patients were women, he personally insisted, as Willis and Sydenham had done two centuries earlier, that hysteria was not solely a female malady, but, on the contrary, could be diagnosed and detected among the male of the species. Hysteria was, he confidently declared, a disorder of the nervous system, not of the female reproductive organs. It was, moreover, as real and as somatic a disease as any of the other neurological catastrophes he had earlier elucidated.

Charcot had been born in humble circumstances, the son of a wagon-maker. He rose to eminence through the competitive examination system that Napoleon had introduced to the French in the aftermath of the Revolution, a poor boy made good. Along the way, he secured a position at the Salpêtrière, a vast warren of buildings on the edge of Paris that Louis XIV had made into "the Versailles of pain," a receptacle for the (female) sweepings of the city: beggars, adulteresses, prostitutes, the depraved, those afflicted with venereal diseases, the senile, and the insane. An appointment to run some of the dilapidated wards in what Charcot himself called this "great emporium of human misery" might not have seemed a stroke of good fortune, but so it proved to be. For the Salpêtrière's inhabitants made up an unrivaled collection of neurological specimens, together constituting what he called "a sort of living pathological museum [*une sorte de Musée patholigique vivant*] whose resources are almost inexhaustible."[1] It was a museum to which Charcot had privileged access, and it was on this foundation that he constructed his career and worldwide fame.

Charcot had been well trained in the clinico-pathological tradition that had emerged in the Paris hospitals in the early nineteenth century, a then-revolutionary approach to disease and debility that emphasized a localized pathology, and the correlation of ante-mortem signs and symptoms with post-mortem findings. Of necessity, this new hospital medicine required a constant supply of patients who would soon turn into corpses, for it was this never-failing availability of previously examined bodies that allowed the comparison of the living and the dead. This inspection in its turn allowed the clinician to uncover the lesions that had produced the earlier signs and symptoms, thus permitting the construction of authoritative portraits of particular diseases. What to the lay outsider must have looked like one of the least desirable portions of Dante's Inferno was for Charcot a living museum of pathology, and, as its specimens ceased breathing, their poor and friendless status ensured that he had at his disposal the means to investigate and catalogue a vast spectrum of neurological complaints. And, since his appointment lasted decades, he could even follow the sometimes remitting and always complex natural history of neurological illnesses over extended periods of time. From a place to store the stigmatized and unwanted, the Salpêtrière was thus transformed into "a Temple of Science."

To be sure, it took talent, energy, ambition, and drive to take advantage of these circumstances, but these Charcot possessed in abundance. Through the 1860s, he and his students labored doggedly at their task. By the end of the decade, Charcot could claim credit for a whole string of diagnostic distinctions and clinical advances. Attending only to his neurological triumphs, he had identified disseminated multiple sclerosis; aphasia; amyotrophic lateral sclerosis (for the French, "Charcot's disease"; for Americans, since the 1930s, Lou Gehrig's disease, after the great baseball player who died from it); locomotor ataxia (a complication of tertiary syphilis, as would become apparent in the early twentieth century); Tourette's syndrome (named for one of Charcot's assistants); Charcot-Marie atrophy; and chorea. These were but the most striking of his accomplishments, a series of scientific triumphs that cemented his reputation at the very peak of neurology, and made his word law. If Charcot diagnosed the patient's disorder, the matter was settled, and it was the vast reservoir of authority he derived from his expertise in these dismal diseases of the nervous system that gave him license to pronounce and pontificate on the puzzles of hysteria/mysteria, and to assert that here was another in the array of largely incurable diseases of the nervous system.

Many French physicians were loathe to admit hysteria to the status of a legitimate disease. Acknowledged as "a wastepaper basket of medicine where one throws otherwise unemployed symptoms,"[2] to use the words of the Parisian alienist Charles Lasègue, it was for many doctors a highly suspect category. In the contemptuous language of another physician at the Salpêtrière, Jules Falret, the women who purported to suffer from hysteria were

> veritable actresses; they do not know a greater pleasure than to deceive…all those with whom they come in touch. The hysterics who exaggerate their convulsive movement…make an equal travesty and exaggeration of the movements of their souls, their ideas, and their acts…in a word, the life of the

> hysteric is nothing but one perpetual falsehood; they affect
> the airs of piety and devotion, and let themselves be taken for
> saints while at the same time abandoning themselves to the
> most shameful actions; and at home, before their husbands
> and children, make the most violent scenes in which they
> employ the coarsest and often most obscene language and
> give themselves up to the most disorderly actions.[3]

Acting, deception, shameful and perpetual falsehood, these are descriptors that are redolent of moral disgust and condemnation, not the neutral tones of the clinician confronting biological infirmity. Charcot, by contrast, was insistent that hysteria was a genuinely organic disorder, a disease rooted firmly in the higher nervous system, and in these respects part of the broader spectrum of neurological disorders.

At first blush, such assertions seem, and must have seemed, paradoxical. Charcot had done more than any of his contemporaries to map out the disorders and lesions of the nervous system, and the tics, the anesthesias, the seizures, and paralyses that were such central elements in hysterical attacks were defined precisely by their failure to correspond to the anatomical realities, the physical topography of the body. Before Charcot, for example, it had been commonplace to confuse the tremblings of the victims of Parkinson's disease with those of multiple sclerosis. Through careful comparison he had distinguished the two, and linked the tremors of multiple sclerosis to distinctive anatomical lesions of the spinal cord that were observable post-mortem. This work involved matching precise clinical observations of patients to what he observed at autopsy, irregular, grey, sclerotic patches that were nonetheless sharply distinguished from adjacent structures and were "disseminated without any apparent rule, and as if at random, over all points of the [spinal] cord"; and then uncovering the distinctive microscopy of the disease. Later, he would correlate similar plaques on the brain to the disorders of vision, speech, and intellect that may manifest themselves as part of the natural history of the disease.

It was precisely on the ability to make increasingly fine diagnostic (and prognostic) distinctions that neurologists' authority rested, for then, as now, virtually all these neurological disasters were incurable. As the man who had done most to establish the foundations on which the emerging specialty rested its claims to expertise, Charcot enjoyed prestige and professional standing that were without peer. His intellectual pre-eminence, together with the near-autocratic power he came to possess over access to elite positions in the French medical establishment, allowed him to stifle most dissent, and secure overt allegiance to his claims about hysteria, at least during his lifetime.

By contrast with those of multiple sclerosis, the patterns of the observed symptoms in cases of hysteria reflected lay and common-sense understandings of how the body was put together, but explicitly contradicted what professional, specialized knowledge had shown those connections and linkages to be. Hysterical deficits were, more often than not, neuroanatomical impossibilities. Yet Charcot invoked and invested his prestige and standing as "the Napoleon of the neuroses" to insist on their bodily reality. They were, he acknowledged, "morbid states, evidently having their seat in the nervous system, which leave in the dead body no material trace that can be discovered." Hysteria did not stand alone in this regard: epilepsy and the choreas (degenerative nervous disorders characterized by spasmodic movements of the face, body, and limbs, and a loss of coordination) also "deny the most penetrating anatomical investigations." All these neurological diseases,

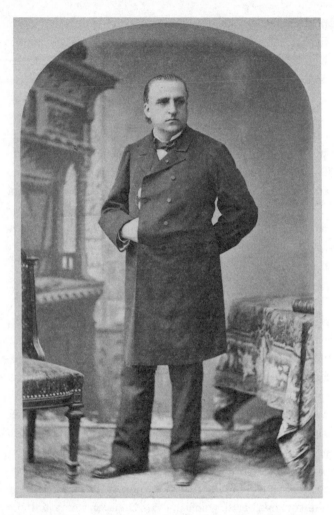

9. Jean-Martin Charcot (1829–93) obviously took his nickname "the Napoleon of the Neuroses" quite seriously. He gave this portrait to his acolyte, Sigmund Freud, with a note in his own hand, on Freud's departure from Paris on February 24, 1886. A precious possession, it was carefully preserved among Freud's effects. (*Freud Museum, London*)

in consequence, "do not present themselves to the mind of the physician with that appearance of solidity, of objectivity, which belong to affections connected with an appreciable organic lesion."[4] And yet, Charcot insisted, they were indeed disorders of the nervous system, just as much as multiple sclerosis and the rest. Hysteria, in particular, which some sought to banish "into the category of the unknown," was the product of an underlying hysterical diathesis, and belonged without question to the same family as the many diseases of the nervous system he had already dissected.

Though his primitive microscopes could detect no lesions on which to pin the disease, hysterical patients, for Charcot, displayed the next best thing: physical stigmata revelatory of the underlying inherited physical inferiority that gave birth to their symptoms. There was an overlooked circularity here: the headaches, the visual problems, the (sometimes migrating) loss of sensation on one side of the body (hemianesthesias), the convulsive fits that resembled (but were clearly not) epileptic seizures, and that Charcot would label "la grande hystérie"—these were at once the signs that signaled the presence of an inherited set of physical deficiencies, and the basis on which hysteria could be diagnosed. Ovarian tenderness, too, marked the female patients out, a sign of the continued hold reflex theory had on Charcot's thinking. Applying pressure on a hysterical woman's ovaries by pushing down on her abdomen could modify the symptoms she displayed, just as, Charcot discovered, squeezing a hysterical male's testicles might provoke changes in his behavior and still greater convulsions. In the case of one 16-year-old girl, for example, pressure on her abdomen in the "ovarian" region had dramatic effects:

Immediately an attack of rhythmic chorea breaks out. The patient remains sitting and her consciousness is preserved. Her head begins suddenly to turn from right to left, and then from left to right, in rhythmic alteration with equal pauses between the individual movements. Simultaneously, the right arm begins going up and down, as a result of which her right hand beats regularly on her knee as though on a drum. The movements of the hand are synchronized with those of the head. Meanwhile the right foot is stamping noisily on the floor. There are approximately 100 beats of the foot and three times as many of the hand in a minute.[5]

Beyond the echoes of reflex theory such examples conjure up, the emphasis on a defective physical constitution was a variation of the theories of degeneration as a cause of crime, alcoholism, violence, and madness. The concept of degeneration was broadly embraced in the last third of the nineteenth century— nowhere more enthusiastically than among asylum doctors, for whom this ideology at once provided a new legitimation for the mental hospital, and an explanation for their failure to deliver on their earlier promises of cure. For Charcot, such notions provided indispensable support for his assertions about hysteria's organicity.

Two factors were of particular importance in directing steadily more of Charcot's attention to the problem of hysteria. First, he was given authority in 1870 over yet another ward in the Salpêtrière, a space for thirty patients where epileptics and hysterics were clustered together, and where, almost by osmosis, the hysterical patients seemed to have acquired a propensity for major fits. Though this was scarcely Charcot's first encounter with either disorder, the combination fascinated him, and drew him away from the study of the scleroses and related disorders, and more and more towards an interest in what he first termed "hystero-epilepsy," and would later dub "la grande hystérie" or "hystérie major." Secondly, there was his late 1870s embrace of "hypnosis," the term James Braid had invented in 1843 in an effort to detoxify the odors of quackery that had enveloped mesmerism. For Charcot, the use of hypnosis led directly to the apotheosis of his Tuesday spectacles, the ever more elaborate display of the pathologies of his hysterical patients that brought him such large and entranced audiences. Earlier in the 1870s, the audience for his lectures had been small and purely professional, some fellow physicians and a handful of interns. His hypnotic séances soon multiplied their numbers many times over, broadening their appeal and attracting a host of the laity.

Again, we seem to enter an Alice-in-Wonderland world. For surely the basis of the hypnotic trance is suggestion, the manipulation of psychological states? Not for Charcot, nor, it should be said, for Braid himself, at least when he initially coined the term. And not for Charcot's British contemporaries, who, like him, claimed that only the biologically susceptible—that is, the hysterical—could be hypnotized. Part of Braid's break with mesmerism, and of his attempt to reclaim the technique for medicine, had been his rejection of Mesmer's doctrine of "animal magnetism," and his insistence that what occurred in hypnosis was a change in cerebral circulation, the provoking of a changed state of the nervous system analogous to what one saw in sleep. It was, he insisted, "merely a simple, speedy, and certain method of throwing the nervous system into a new condition..."[6] For Charcot, and his counterparts across the Channel, it was a bit more than that: it was a technique that could work only when practiced upon the defective—indeed, to be hypnotizable was to reveal oneself as a hysteric, to make manifest an underlying diseased state of the entire organism.

Hypnotism and hysteria, in Michael Clark's felicitous summary, were "closely related states of mental and moral [and I would add, physical] degeneracy."[7] The inherited weakness created a prodigious predisposition to the disease, which was then typically triggered by trauma—an accident, violence, perhaps even by the presence of another hysteric, when the hysterical manifestations might multiply and travel from patient to patient, in a veritable epidemic of mass hysteria.

At their core, Charcot's dazzling displays of his hysterical patients were flamboyant, dramatic occasions. The Great Man was, as Ruth Harris notes, "ruthlessly insensitive to the pain and anguish of his patients, and so enamoured of his scientific mission that he dispensed with ethical proprieties when presenting them to the public."[8] Those who were at the center of a particular week's lecture were brought on to the stage, to be examined, poked and prodded, hypnotized, all-but-anatomized by the professor himself, their foibles and physical contortions made the centerpiece of the week's entertainment and instruction.

Sometimes, the drama had a rapid and satisfying conclusion. There was the case of Henriette A., for example, a laundress whose hysteria, like that of many of Charcot's patients, seemed to have its origins in a traumatic incident; in this case she had suffered a glancing blow on the head from a falling bookshelf. The accident left her agitated but apparently unhurt, but a day later, she had suffered a fall, which was soon followed by a developing paralysis of her right arm. In Charcot's hands, the upshot was an almost instantaneous cure, a piece of magic carried out in front of an enthusiastic crowd, and climaxing with Henriette prancing "round among the audience vigorously shaking them by the [right] hand, desirous of proving how real was the recovery they had just witnessed."[9]

But this was a simple case. Others proved far more challenging, and incapable of real amendment. As he had earlier done with cases of multiple sclerosis, Charcot was determined to explore the natural history of hysteria, its characteristic forms and its development over time. All his efforts to localize hysteria in the morgue met with frustration, so he turned to the shifting kaleidoscope of symptoms with which his parade of patients provided him, and sought to produce order from the apparent chaos. A classificatory schema, a sequence of stages through which all patients passed, these were what he thought he detected, and what in reality he manufactured.

Hysteria, Charcot pronounced, had four distinct stages, "four periods [that] succeeded each other in the complete attack with mechanical regularity." There was first an *epileptoide* period, where the patient suffered fits. In the next phase, the "period of contortions and *grands mouvements*," as its name implies, the patient engaged in dramatic physical displays, often accompanied by cries and shrieks, and culminating in some cases in the adoption of an *arc-en-cercle* position, in which the patient bent backwards into a seemingly impossible contortion, with only the back of the head and the heels still touching the ground. Charcot also referred to these episodes as *clownisme*. Then, especially in female patients, there was a phase where the patient adopted *attitudes passionelles*, posing as if being crucified, or in the throes of erotic ecstasy.[10]

In the final or terminal phase of delirium, the patient might experience hallucinations or delusions, which gradually subsided. "What I want to emphasize," Charcot insisted in 1882, "is that in the [hysterical] fit, nothing is left to chance, that to the contrary everything unfolds according to the rules, which are always the same and characterize what we see in outpatients as well as inpatients; they are valid for all countries, for all epochs,

1ᵉʳᵉ PÉRIODE — PÉRIODE ÉPILEPTOÏDE

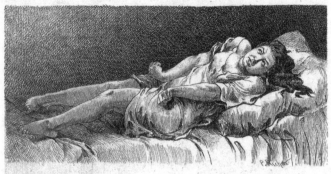

Phase d'immobilité Tonique
ou Tétanisme

10. The first phase of Charcot's *grand hystérie*. The patient, having suffered a seizure, is locked into a tonic immobility, arms rigid, nightgown rucked up. (*Wellcome Library, London*)

for all races, and are, in short, universal."[11] And, of course, it was that universality, that regularity, that lent weight to his contention that hysteria was an organic disease of the nervous system—except that the regularity and the universalism were manufactured, socially constructed by Charcot's assistants and their pliable specimens, though the *mise en scène* took place behind Charcot's back, and in all probability without his knowledge.

Charcot was, however, fully conscious of the possibility of simulation, and aware that those who rejected his claims about the reality of hysteria saw the patients as malingerers and fakes. "Here is an element," he acknowledged, "that we meet with at each step…of this neurosis, and which throws (there is no use in denying it) a certain amount of disfavor on the studies which are connected with it. But," he went on, "is it really as difficult

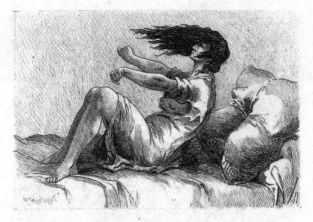

Fig. 1.   Phase des grands mouvements

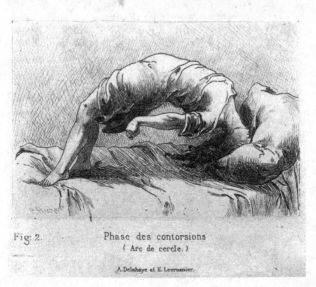

Fig. 2.   Phase des contorsions
(Arc de cercle.)

A.Delahaye et E. Lecrosnier.

11. *Clownisme,* Charcot's second stage of a hysterical attack. The bottom plate shows the characteristic *arc-en-cercle* adopted by many of his patients. (*Wellcome Library, London*)

3ᴱ PÉRIODE — PÉRIODE DES ATTITUDES PASSIONNELLES

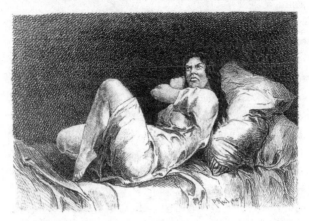

Fig. 1   Phase triste

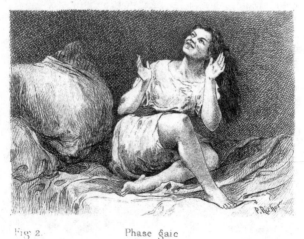

Fig. 2.   Phase gaie

A.Delahaye et E.Lecrosnier.

12. *Attitudes passionelles*, the third phase of *grand hystérie*. Engravings based on one of many photographic studies of the female patients who made up Charcot's circus. (*Wellcome Library, London*)

as some appear to believe, to discern the real symptomatology from the imaginary? By no means."[12] One could, as Charcot proceeded to do, devise experiments to demonstrate the distinction. Hysterics in the cataleptic phase, for example, might keep an arm extended for an extraordinary amount of time, and instruments could be used to trace the least oscillations of the outstretched limb, documenting a difference between the true hysteric and the person who was merely simulating the disorder. "A hundred other examples," he triumphantly concluded, "might be invoked which would only show that the simulation, which is talked about so much when hysteria and allied affections are under consideration, is, in the actual state of our knowledge, only a bugbear, before which the fearful and novice alone are stopped."[13]

Charcot had his favorites, those who returned time and again to put on multiple, often increasingly elaborate, performances. None was more famous than Blanche Wittman, the queen of hysterics, a performer who luxuriated in her role. Perhaps the most famous single image of a hysterical patient is an 1887 painting by André Brouillet that captures Charcot presenting Blanche, his pet hysteric, to members of his neurological service. She swoons over the outstretched arm of his assistant, Joseph Babinski, her pelvis thrust forward, her breasts barely covered by her blouse and pointing suggestively toward the professor, her head twisted to the side and her face contorted in what looks like the throes of orgasm. (Freud kept a copy of this painting, which dates from 1887, in his study in Vienna, and again in London.)

Wittman was admitted to the Salpêtrière in 1878, and remained there for some sixteen years, performing on command. After her discharge, she became Marie Curie's laboratory assistant, and eventually was poisoned by the radium she was working with. In consequence, both legs and her left arm

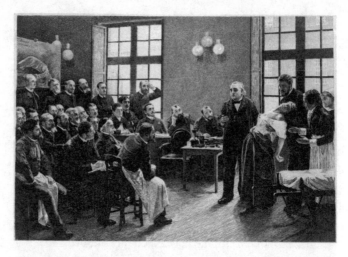

13. Blanche Wittman (1863–1913), the "queen of hysterics," in the archetypical portrait of Charcot demonstrating a case of hysteria before a rapt audience. (*Wellcome Library, London*)

had to be amputated. Then there was Augustine, admitted to the Salpêtrière in 1875 at 15½,

> tall, well-developed (neck a bit thick, ample breasts, under-arms and pubis covered with hair), with a determined tone and bearing, temperamental, noisy. No longer behaving in the least like a child, she looks almost like a full-grown woman, and yet she has never menstruated. She was admitted for paralysis of sensation in her right arm, preceded by pains in her lower right abdomen.[14]

She had, we now know, been threatened with a razor and raped by her mother's lover when only 13, and sexually attacked by other men in her neighborhood. Once in the hospital, she was stripped and displayed, physically and emotionally laid bare, photographed incessantly in diaphanous and revealing

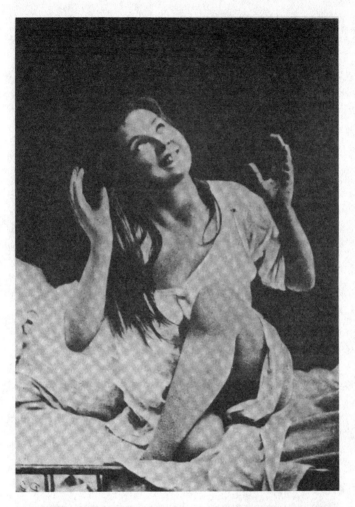

14. Augustine, before she stole away from the Salpêtrière. Frequently caught by the camera lens in erotic poses, here she poses half naked in a state of *extase*, or ecstasy.

hospital gowns for the multi-volume Catalogue of images that constituted the *Iconographie* and the *Nouvelle Iconographie* of the Salpêtrière, Augustine would play a starring role in the circus for five years, till, one day in September 1880, she abruptly stole away, disguised (and this sealed her status as a Surrealist and then a feminist icon) as a man, never to be heard from again.

But the supporting cast grew ever more numerous, and the audience steadily larger and more heterogeneous. Axel Munthe has provided us with a vivid reconstruction of the scene, one he himself observed and participated in. Out beyond the stage, "the huge amphitheatre was filled to the last place with a multi-coloured audience drawn from tout Paris, authors, journalists, leading actors and actresses, fashionable demimondaines"—all gathered for the show. Now came the performers, the grey-coated, sombre Charcot, the master of ceremonies for the proceedings, and then the women who would do his bidding, apparently under the influence of the hypnotic trance:

> Some of them smelt with delight a bottle of ammonia when told it was rose water, others would eat a piece of charcoal when presented to them as chocolate. Another would crawl on all fours on the floor, barking furiously when told she was a dog, flap her arms as if trying to fly when turned into a pigeon, lift her skirts with a shriek of terror when a glove was thrown at her feet with a suggestion of being a snake. Another would walk with a top hat in her arms rocking it to and fro and kissing it tenderly when told it was a baby."[15]

The masculine dominance, the foolishness and frailty of the female, both were decisively on display.

The *Iconographies*, the collections of photographs of the performers who made up the circus, circulated widely and disseminated the Charcotian vision of hysteria to an audience who could only virtually witness the Parisian scene. They did much to fix the image of hysteria in the public mind, and perhaps to spread suggestively what purported to be neutral, naturalistic recordings of a neuropathic disorder. The photograph (at least before the age of digital manipulation) carried the illusion of providing the truth, a direct and unmediated portrait or even a mirror of nature, the instantaneous representation of what passed before the lens of the camera. But the limitations of lighting, and the technical requirements of picture-taking with wet collodion plates, or even the later silver gelatino-bromide coating, made for long exposures, sometimes as long as twenty minutes per plate. Perhaps appropriately, given that Charcot's posthumous critics (whom, as we shall see, included even— in fact, especially—his collaborators and protégés) viewed his clinical demonstrations as fraudulent, the "objective" photographs that recorded the pathologies were themselves necessarily staged, posed, and manufactured constructions whose status as "facts" is as slippery as the live demonstrations they purport to record.

Charcot was not alone in exploiting his patients, in treating them as so many specimens rather than as suffering human beings. The disdain and the callousness were a feature of the whole clinico-pathological tradition, something that American medical students visiting Paris for instruction viewed with dismay as early as the 1830s. As feminist historians focused their attentions on hysteria as a female complaint, and perhaps the product, as some of them speculated, of an inchoate, inarticulate protest against the roles in which Victorian women were imprisoned, Charcot's serial exploitations of these poor creatures, his willingness to expose them repeatedly to the prurient gaze of his audience at whatever cost to their emotional well-being, drew fierce criticism and reproof. But those same moral failings were visible to Charcot's contemporaries, and were the subject of bitter commentary, even from literary figures such as Tolstoy and de Maupassant. A Madame Renooz, in the pages of the *Revue scientifique des femmes*, protested about his "sort of vivisection of women under the pretext of studying a disease for which he knows neither the cause nor the treatment."[16] And across the Channel, another critic condemned the

> disgusting experiments practiced on lunatics and hysterical patients in the Salpêtrière. The nurses drag these unfortunate women, notwithstanding their cries and resistance, before men who make them fall into catalepsy. They play on these organisms...on which the experiment strains the nervous system and aggravates the morbid conditions, as if it were an instrument...One of my friends told me that she...had seen a doctor of great reputation make one unhappy patient pass, without transition, from a celestial beatitude to a condition of infamous sensualment. And this before a company of literary men and men of the world.[17]

And yet Charcot, as the feminist historian Elaine Showalter acknowledges, cannot be easily typecast as a crude misogynist, for he adopted liberal positions by the standards of his time on women's rights, and his students and externs included women training for the medical profession. Moreover, one of Charcot's more striking departures from the conventional wisdom of his time had been his insistence that hysteria was not just a female disease. Earlier proponents of a neuropathic etiology for hysteria, such as Willis and Sydenham, had made this point in the late seventeenth century, but reflex theory had created a new way of re-emphasizing the connections between women's reproductive organs, their brains, and their propensity to be hysterical.

Thomas Laycock, writing in 1840, had drawn upon such ideas to reassert that "hysteria is peculiar to females" because it is "the nervous system of the woman which is implicated in these affections."[18] And some decades later, Beard's invention of neurasthenia, while not precluding men from being diagnosed with hysteria, had created an alternative diagnostic label many physicians used disproportionately for men.

Charcot, on the other hand, controversially insisted on emphasizing that hysteria afflicted males as well as females. His colleague Pierre Briquet of the Hôpital de la Charité in Paris had made similar claims in 1859, arguing against those who had used reflex theory to relink hysteria to women's reproductive organs, and Charcot acknowledged his debt to Briquet many times in lectures and in print. Charcot had opened a ward for hysterical males at the Salpêtrière, in 1882, the first accommodation for men that the vast hospital had ever made, and male patients had also attended his out-patient clinics from 1878 onwards. Beginning in the 1880s, perhaps a quarter of his published discussions of hysteria focused on men, and his contradiction of the traditional view that hysteria was a female disorder drew widespread attention.

Although the claim that masculine hysterics existed was certainly not new, generally such cases had been ignored or marginalized. Often, when they were recognized as such, hysterical males had been dismissed as effeminate, sedentary, and studious. Many of Charcot's male patients, by contrast, were drawn from the laboring classes and were muscular, virile men—in his words "vigoreux, solide, non énervé par la culture."[19] They included train drivers, plumbers, bakers, blacksmiths, and the like. Earlier generations, Charcot insisted, had simply misdiagnosed such cases, whereas modern medical science (in whose vanguard, of course, he stood) had finally grasped their true nature. As with his female hysterics, Charcot emphasized the neuropathic origins of these men's disorders, and, in parallel fashion, it was the men's hemianesthesias and their paralyses, their contractures and their seizures, rather than their psychological disturbances, that were the primary focus of his attentions. Just as American neurologists had dismissed the efforts of gynecologists to trespass on neurological territory, so these emphases in Charcot's theorizing not so coincidentally cut the ground out from under French gynecologists who were tempted to endorse ovariotomies as a cure for hysteria.

Charcot's emphasis on the prevalence of hysteria among men of the artisanal and working classes reflected a more general way in which his writings on hysteria departed from most prior orthodoxy. Where standard discussions had tended to stress the connection between nervous disorders and affluence, and this claim was as clear in Cheyne's remarks on the English malady as in Beard's commentary on American nervousness, Charcot's female patients at the Salpêtrière were almost all drawn from the lower orders. For both sexes, therefore, he was led to acknowledge that previous discussions of hysteria's social location had gone badly astray. "We must not forget," he commented with some asperity,

> that the psychological constitution [of the working class] is fundamentally the same as ours, and that, perhaps even more than other people, they are subjected to the destructive effects of painful moral emotions, of anxieties related to the material difficulties of life, to the depressing influence of the exaggerated effect of physical forces…In addition, we should remember that neuropathic heredity is scarcely the exclusive privilege of the wealthy in life. It extends its reach to the working class as to everywhere else.

Hysteria, not surprisingly, may thus "be observed on a grand scale among the workers and artisans, by those the least favored by fate and who scarcely know anything other than hard manual labor."[20]

Among patients with an inherited hysterical diathesis, it took only a precipitating event to bring about a full-blown hysterical attack. Alcohol was one such precipitant, especially among the lower orders. But so were industrial accidents and other traumatic incidents, railway accidents being one of the most common of these, both for Charcot, and for those trying to trace the etiology of the disorder elsewhere in Europe and North America. Here, Charcot verged on accepting the notion that ideas and emotions could be sufficient to precipitate a breakdown, though it was a model of how hysteria might materialize that he could never fully bring himself to accept. Understanding hysteria in terms of the "conversion" of the psychological into the physical was a move that would be left to others.

One of the hallmarks of the French academic system, and in many ways one of its great weaknesses, was its hierarchical and hyper-centralized character. (In this respect it mimicked the larger society that had spawned and supported it.) Those who stood at the head of the system could lord it over all beneath them, and no one more so than Charcot. Like many a poor boy made good, he liked nothing better than to mingle with the rich and the powerful.

His marriage to a wealthy widow, combined with the robust clinical income secured by his growing reputation, allowed him to purchase both a villa in the affluent suburb of Neuilly-sur-Seine and an elegant mansion, 217 Boulevard Saint-Germain, and to furnish both with tapestries, paintings, rare books, antiques, even stained-glass windows. His bookshelves, for example, were modeled on those found in Florence in the library of the Medicis in the Convent of San Lorenzo, and his collection of classical and

Renaissance art provided him with an array of paintings depicting the visions and ecstasies of saints, portraits he delighted in reinterpreting as instances of undiagnosed hysteria. Charcot's intellectual fortunes were in important ways linked to the fiercely anti-clerical politics of the Third Republic. His chair of nervous diseases, for example, had been pushed through the National Assembly by his prominent political friend Léon Gambetta. How better to return the favor, to tweak the forces of religious reaction, and to discredit the most sacred characters of Christian martyrdom, than by declaring them to be a collection of specimens of mental pathology, mere deluded hysterics?

In the splendid setting of his city mansion, Charcot held regular soirées on Tuesdays after his public lectures, glittering affairs that brought together writers and poets, journalists and architects, statesmen and scientists, the occasional cardinal and the elite of the medical profession. Such figures were powerful allies, adding to the immense authority Charcot had already derived from his chair at the Paris medical faculty and from his increasingly global prominence. By the 1880s it was plausibly asserted that all appointments to the medical faculty required his imprimatur, an influence that he was not in the least shy about exercising.

What made this concentration of power the more dangerous was that Charcot was notoriously thin-skinned—allergic, not just to criticism, but even to minor forms of dissent among his underlings. To court the professor's displeasure was to invite severe damage to one's prospects, even professional ruin. Those who feared or had felt his wrath might take their revenge through the traditional subterranean tactics of the weak: damaging the careers of his protégés, for instance, when they could do so without fear of detection (as when Charles Bouchard, a rival neurologist, placed the young Joseph Babinski at the bottom of the *aggrégation* list, ensuring that the most talented French neurologist of his generation could never achieve the rank of professor); but seldom or never daring to confront him directly. In the words of Léon Daudet, the son of one of Charcot's closest friends, the great professor "could not stand contradiction, however small. If someone dared to contradict his theories, he became ferocious and mean and did all he could to wreck the career of the imprudent man unless he retracted and apologized."[21] On a broader canvas, he was envious of others' successes, and, according to the Goncourt brothers, showed "a ferocious resentment against those who declined invitations to his receptions."[22]

The salutary correctives that close associates, or even independent rivals, might have on the great man's wilder fancies were thus notable for their absence. Charcot found himself surrounded by yes-men and mediocrities, and those too frightened to speak out. Not only did this heighten the danger that his views might become entrenched in increasingly dubious and indefensible positions, but, as the sycophantic scurried to secure his favor, it actually encouraged them to stage performances for his benefit—fraudulent events that lent apparent intellectual support to increasingly suspect claims. In the final years before his death, even Charcot had begun to question whether there was not indeed a strong psychological component to hysteria, though for the most part he remained convinced of its organic roots. (In any event, it was an article of faith with Charcot that the realm of the psychological would ultimately prove reducible to cerebral physiology.) With his demise, however, the whole Charcotian edifice came rapidly crashing down.

In tribute to the great man, there was a project to publish his complete works, but it was soon abandoned and never revived, with only nine of a projected twenty-six volumes ever appearing in print. His long-cowed pupils now dared to voice their dissent, and men like Babinski and Déjerine (who succeeded to Charcot's chair in 1911) were soon distancing themselves from the legacy of their *maître*, and denying the reality of the dramas they had once had so large a hand in staging. Babinski made his intellectual break with his patron clear by moving, in 1901, to do away with the label of "hysteria" altogether, and to replace it with a term of his own coinage, "pithiatism." Déjerine waited only a little longer. "It now seems certain," he said, almost two decades after his patron was safely in the grave, "that the crises delineated by this description [*la grande hystérie*] are nothing other than coaching [*dressage*] and imitation."[23] Axel Munthe was more biting yet:

> these stage performances of the Salpêtrière before the public of Tout Paris were nothing but an absurd farce, a hopeless muddle of truth and cheating. Some of these subjects were no doubt real somnambulists faithfully carrying out in a waking state the various suggestions made to them during sleep—posthypnotic suggestions. Many of them were mere frauds, knowing quite well what they were expected to do, delighted to perform their various tricks in public, cheating both doctors and audience with the amazing cunning of the *hystériques*. They were always ready to *piquer une attaque* of Charcot's *grande hystérie, arc-en-ciel* and all, or to exhibit his famous three stages of hypnotism: lethargy, catalepsy, somnambulism, all invented by the Master...[24]

All that for decades had seemed so solid melted into air. The very term "hysteria" vanished with astonishing rapidity from the French scene, and the epicenter of the hysterical imperium moved hundreds of miles to the east and south, to the hothouse, sexualized atmosphere of *fin-de-siècle* Vienna. As early as 1900, Charcot's star had firmly set.

VII

FREUDIAN HYSTERICS

On October 13, 1885, the Orient Express, which had then been in operation a scant two years, pulled into the Gare de l'Est in Paris at the end of its long journey from Austria. A bearded 29-year-old man descended from his carriage and joined the crowds moving towards the Boulevard de Strasbourg. Poor but ambitious, he was making one last desperate throw of the dice before facing the grim prospect of exile, perhaps to the United States, a country he regarded as "a hopeless place for science" and one he would later dismiss as "gigantic, but a gigantic mistake."[1]

Our weary traveller had trained in medicine in Vienna, where his prior efforts to build an academic career in zoology, then in physiology, and finally in neuro-anatomy had ended in disappointment. Worse yet, he was fleeing a growing controversy provoked by his therapeutic experiments with cocaine, a substance he had claimed was a wonder drug, but one that others found led to addiction, destruction of the personality, and death. His private life was equally messy. Engaged since 1882, he was desperate to marry. Yet it seemed he could do so only by abandoning his scientific ambitions and settling down to a mundane, perhaps maddening, existence as a practicing clinician. At the last, only the forceful intervention of his mentor, Ernst Brücke, had enabled him to secure a small grant to support him for six months in Paris, where he planned to work under the great Jean-Martin Charcot, who was then at the height of his fame.

Even with this prospect in front of him, Sigmund Freud looked at a bleak future, and his first weeks in Paris did little to relieve the gloom. Charcot's reputation drew would-be neurologists to Paris like iron filings to a magnet, and nothing enabled the young Austrian to stand out from the crowd of professionals jostling for the great man's attention and favors. Or, rather, nothing did until Freud conceived the idea of putting himself forward as someone who could translate Charcot's latest lectures into German. Once his offer had been accepted, Freud found himself inside the charmed circle, at least to the extent of being invited to the soirées held on Tuesdays at Charcot's mansion on the Boulevard Saint-Germain. And Freud was as good as his word. Though by his own admission his spoken French was atrocious, he produced a German translation of the third volume of Charcot's *Leçons sur les maladies du système nerveux* that appeared in print even before the French original was published.

The mark of Charcot's favor made Freud a devoted disciple. Yet even still, his stay in Paris lasted a bare four and a half months. Charcot was ill for some of that time, and Freud also took a two-week vacation at Christmas to spend time with his fiancée, Martha Bernays. Yet the Parisian circus that he experienced at first hand had made a profound impression, entirely reorienting his intellectual horizons. As he wrote to Martha on November 24, within weeks of settling in Paris, "Charcot, who is one of the greatest of physicians and a man whose common sense borders on genius, is simply wrecking all of my aims and opinions. I sometimes come out of his lectures as from out of Notre Dame, with an entirely new idea about perfection."[2] In February of the new year, Freud returned to Vienna with all the enthusiasm of a convert, bent upon enlightening the Viennese medical elite about Charcot's discoveries concerning hysteria and his use of hypnosis.

Freud seems to have been oblivious to the impression his bumptiousness and his embrace of a French rival would have on his superiors. A lecture before his elders at the Viennese Medical Association was greeted with little enthusiasm. In a forum that was supposed to be devoted to relaying original scientific discoveries of one's own, Freud proffered only a warmed-over version of what he had observed at the Salpêtrière. His claim that Charcot's emphasis on male hysteria was novel was roundly dismissed by colleagues, who proceeded to recall their own encounters with male hysterics decades earlier. And, while Charcot's institutional power and ruthlessness had caused the French medical establishment to drop its long hostility towards hypnosis, no such transformation of attitudes had occurred in the German-speaking world. Theodor Meynert, in particular, a dominant figure in Freud's world, was scathingly dismissive of hypnosis as nothing more than quackery. Freud's espousal of the technique did nothing to commend him to his superiors.

Making matters worse, over the last half of the 1880s, Charcot's claims about hypnosis and its relationship to hysteria were coming under sustained assault even in France. To be sure, the attacks came from the periphery, from the provincial city of Nancy in eastern France, and the Napoleon of the neuroses must have felt they posed little threat to his entrenched authority. But Charcot's claims that only a minority of people, those who were afflicted with an inherited neuropathic taint, were vulnerable to hypnosis, and that the hypnotized passed through a regular series of predictable stages were weakened to the point of collapse by Bernheim's repeated demonstrations that neither was empirically so. Validation of the upstart Frenchman's claims by others made a mockery of Charcot's assertions, a viewpoint that was embraced even in Paris following the great man's death in 1892. For many, the upshot was a renewed conviction that hypnosis was the product of "mere" suggestion (rather than, as Charcot had argued, a primarily physiological process), and thus a species of self-delusion, charlatanry, and fraud. The spread of such views may well have prompted Freud to reconsider his own therapeutic investment in hypnosis, a technique he had never truly mastered, and one that by the mid-1890s he would largely abandon.

Freud's return to Vienna and to clinical practice brought his long engagement to a close. Marriage, however, soon brought a parade of children, six of them by 1896, adding substantially to his financial burdens. His private practice in these years was devoted to neurological patients, particularly children with cerebral palsy, but custom was slow to arrive. Such as they were, his clients included a number of cases of indeterminate, "functional" origin, "hysterics," albeit not necessarily of the dramatic sort he had seen in Paris. It was a pattern familiar to many an aspiring neurologist on both sides of the Atlantic, for whom hysterics were an indispensable source of income. These he treated with the standard weapons in the neurologist's repertoire: massage, hydrotherapeutics, electricity, and the rest cure.

In Freud's tenuous circumstances, an important source of patient referrals was a fellow physician many years his senior, Josef Breuer, a colleague Freud had first encountered in Brücke's laboratory. Breuer had developed a large and lucrative practice among Vienna's Jewish *haute bourgeoisie*, a clientele that made him a wealthy man. As his workload grew, he referred some of the overflow to Freud. Periodically, he also relieved the younger man's financial worries with small loans, and the two men grew personally close.

As long ago as 1880, Breuer had treated one particularly remarkable case of hysteria, Bertha Pappenheim, a woman who would become famous to posterity as Anna O. It was a treatment that continued till June of 1882. Bertha/Anna's disturbances were legion. They had surfaced after the sheltered young woman had spent many months nursing her dying father. Her symptoms were dramatic: trance-like states, hallucinations, spasms of coughing, sleeplessness, a refusal to eat or drink, a rigid paralysis of the extremities on the right side of her body, severely disturbed vision, outbreaks of uncontrollable anger, a failure to recognize those around her, and finally a failure of language—first a deterioration of her German, and then an inability to speak or comprehend anything but English, her native language remaining unintelligible to her for eighteen months. Breuer's treatment of her involved frequent and prolonged encounters on a regular basis. According to his account, he eventually found that, by talking with her about her symptoms and, more importantly, by tracing them back to traumatic scenes in her past, they could be made to disappear, the catharsis proving profoundly therapeutic. It was the patient herself who dubbed this "the talking cure."

Such "cures," Breuer acknowledged, required exhaustive (and exhausting) efforts. Bertha/Anna had a remarkable memory, which proved a double-edged sword. Tackling her hearing difficulties alone required sifting, in reverse chronological order, through 303 separate instances when these dysfunctions had materialized. On and on the process went, till the final recalcitrant symptoms—a paralysis of her right arm and her inability to speak her native language—were relieved when she recalled hallucinating about a black snake poised to strike the bedridden father she was tending to, and being unable to move her arm until it occurred to her to recite a prayer in English. The event recalled, the paralysis abruptly vanished, and she was once more able to converse in German.

These dramatic events were frequently the object of Breuer and Freud's conversations, beginning in November 1882. Subsequent scholarship has demolished Breuer's assertions that Bertha/Anna was cured by his ministrations. On the contrary, not long after Breuer abruptly ceased treating her, she was institutionalized by her family at the Sanatorium Bellevue in Kreuzlingen, Switzerland, where she remained for more than three and a half months, still exhibiting a multitude of hysterical symptoms, as well as being addicted to morphine (an aspect of Breuer's treatment of her he never acknowledged in print). Freud himself would eventually claim, in a conversation with his disciple Ernest Jones, that Breuer's therapeutic efforts were terminated abruptly when he discovered that his patient harbored erotic longings for her therapist, longings that expressed themselves in the form of a phantom pregnancy. But this story, too, we now know was fictitious. Instead, Bertha/Anna was re-institutionalized on at least three more occasions in the 1880s, and continued for years after her alleged cure to experience hallucinations and to manifest the whole panoply of her hysterical symptoms, till she finally "recovered" in the early 1890s, a decade after she had ceased being Breuer's patient.

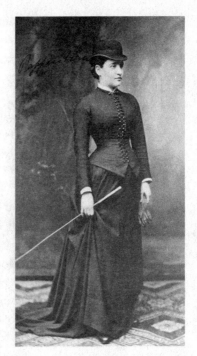

15. Breuer's patient "Anna O.," or Bertha Pappenheim (1859–1936) as seen in 1882. This photograph was taken at the Sanatorium Bellevue at Kreuzlingen, where she was confined as a mental patient. In later life, Pappenheim became a prominent social worker, author, and feminist, no thanks to the talking cure she helped to invent.

All these revelations about Anna O.'s true history were to remain hidden, however, for nearly a century. The myth of her cure through talk therapy would in the meantime circulate and recirculate, and come to form the foundation of a radically novel approach to the treatment and understanding of hysteria. Three years after his return from Paris, Freud himself began employing hypnosis and the cathartic method on a series of his own female patients, beginning with a patient he referred to only as Frau Emmy von N., moving then to Fräulein Elizabeth von R. (his first full-length analysis of hysteria), and then to the cases of Miss Lucy R., Katherina, and Frau Cäcilie M. (about the last of whom he generally sustained a discreet silence, no doubt because of her elevated social status). Like Breuer, he asserted that the process produced results:

> we found, to our great surprise at first, that *each individual hysterical symptom immediately and permanently disappeared when we had succeeded in bringing clearly to light the memory of the event by which it was provoked and in arousing its accompanying affect, and when the patient had described that event in the greatest possible detail and had put the affect into words.*[3]

At length, and primarily at Freud's insistence, the two men's shared experiences prompted them to write a joint monograph on hysteria. A preliminary communication on the subject appeared in 1893, and was followed by the publication two years later of their book *Studies on Hysteria*, to which Freud contributed four lengthy discussions of patients he had treated. To great dramatic effect, a handful of case reports (Anna O. first amongst them) was used to legitimate their theory and treatment. Freud, in particular, wrote his account in the form of a series of psychologically charged vignettes that read, in his own words, "like short stories and that, as one might say,…lack the serious stamp of science"—a discomforting reality that he explained away with the consoling thought that "the nature of the subject is responsible for this, rather than any preference of my own."[4] "*Hysterics,*" Breuer and Freud concluded, "*suffer mainly from reminiscences,*"[5] memories that lingered in repressed form in the unconscious, only to return to the surface with a vengeance years later in the disguised form of symptoms.

Charcot's patients had been drawn in substantial numbers from the ranks of the poor, and his etiological account of the origins of hysteria had placed a correspondingly heavy emphasis on degeneration as the source of their troubles. Freud's and Breuer's patients, by contrast, were privileged and affluent, ill-disposed to being told that they were biologically inferior. Small wonder that Freud warned of the need to abandon "the theoretical prejudice that we are dealing with the abnormal brains of *dégénérés* and *déséquilibrés*."[6] Like Cheyne before them, Breuer and Freud emphasized that hysteria was rather a sign of superiority, the province of the educated, the successful, the well-to-do, the desired, and the desirable. "Hysteria of the severest kind," Freud insisted, "can exist in conjunction with gifts of the richest and most original kind."[7]

It was, as the obese diet doctor had discovered more than a century and a half earlier, a formula that flattered the sensibilities of the hysterical, and did much to increase the clientele of the medics espousing it—which was fortunate, since self-evidently only the rich could afford to indulge in so intensive and extensive a therapy. Frau Cäcilie M., for instance, was twice blessed: born a baroness, and married into still another fortune, this querulous hypochondriac spent the last thirty-three years of her life making various doctors dance to her tunes. For six years, Freud was summoned for daily or twice-daily consultations about her moodiness and hallucinations, obsessions and torments, irritations and anxieties, pains that prevented her walking, and various hysterical conversions that transmuted past experiences into present physical ailments through symbolic association, all of which he sought to trace back to their original traumas—a process that appeared to produce the most intense sufferings in his hypersensitive patient; and a steady stream of fees into the needy Freud's pocket.

By the time their book appeared, it seems that Freud was already falling out with Breuer, and he subsequently claimed

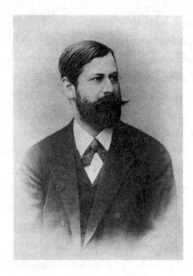

16. Sigmund Freud (1856–1939)
in 1891, four years before the
appearance of *Studies on Hysteria*.
(*Wellcome Library, London*)

that he had already largely lost his faith in the hypnotic and
cathartic techniques their writings recommended. Hysteria,
Freud had concluded, would not yield so readily to the recapitu-
lation of the past. Cathartic sessions might indeed relieve some
hysterical symptoms, but the relief they supplied was only temporary. A more complex approach to the underlying trauma
was required, and it was one that Freud now moved to develop.

There was the question, of course, of the nature of that
trauma. Both men claimed to emphasize the psychological in
their accounts. Breuer, indeed, promised: "In what follows, little
mention will be made of the brain and none whatever of mol-
ecules. Psychical processes will be dealt with in the language
of psychology."[8] In reality, however, he does no such thing.
His text instead emphasizes "intracerebral excitations," and, in
drawing parallels between the nervous system and electrical

installations, he implicitly engages in a reductionism with which Freud would already have been familiar. Charcot, too, in his later years, had increasingly acknowledged the psychological, and had then sought to square his use of such language with his somatic account of hysteria by implying that all things psychological were in reality no more than the surface manifestations of underlying neurological events, what Hughlings Jackson referred to as psychophysical parallelism.

Freud in private was wrestling with this vexed question. He saw that Charcot and Breuer had "solved" this problem by word magic, and that more than vague gestures towards psychophysical parallelism would be required to provide an adequate translation of events at one level into the mechanisms operative at another. But his "project for a scientific psychology," to which he devoted endless hours before and after the publication of *Studies on Hysteria*, and the occasion of multiple written but unpublished drafts, became for him a biological blind alley. At length he set the enterprise to one side as insoluble, indeed itself "a kind of madness." As he confessed in a letter to the Berlin general practitioner Wilhelm Fliess, in November 1895, "I no longer understand the state of mind in which I hatched the psychology."[9] A chemical or physiological account of mental phenomena might ultimately be discovered, but not by him.

Meantime, his case reports about the women he had treated for hysteria had unabashedly stressed the psychological. That provided much of their contemporary and their lasting appeal to a broader audience than his fellow specialists. So did a series of as yet only tantalizing hints of the sexual etiology of hysterical symptoms, for this was a doctrine concerning which Freud himself remained somewhat unsure at this stage. His patients' symptoms, it seemed, were defenses against "*strangulated affect*"[10] that they had somehow sought to suppress, but the nature of those murdered memories, and quite how their repression contributed to the psychopathology of these hysterical women, were yet to be fully worked out. Past events were bound up with undischarged emotions or affect, and years later those stored-up emotions produced pathologies, pathologies that might be alleviated by reliving (or "abreacting") the original experience—but only if the patient's mysterious "amnesia" for the precipitating event could somehow be overcome.

One way of overcoming that unwillingness or inability to cooperate with treatment was to utilize hypnosis. An alternative, with which Freud briefly flirted, was to find ways to make his patients "concentrate," perhaps by applying physical pressure to the forehead. Still another, and this was the approach that ultimately came to dominate and form the very center of psychoanalytic practice, was to allow the patient to "free associate," to speak freely whatever manifested itself in his or her consciousness, and thereby, over time and inadvertently, as it were, to reveal what lay beneath the surface, locked away in unconscious levels of mental activity by what he postulated was a vigilant internal censor. For "free" associations eventually ran up against internally generated roadblocks, forms of repression through which the conscious mind kept secrets from itself, but at the price of converting what it repressed into symptoms. Freud's task, as he saw it, was to comprehend the basis of these internal psychological conflicts, to pry open the patient's defenses, to make the unconscious conscious. Or, rather, to guide the patient to accomplish these tasks, thereby achieving a lasting rearrangement of his or her mental furniture.

By the early 1890s, Breuer had abandoned hysteria as a focus of his practice and as an intellectual puzzle. He acknowledged when the second edition of their monograph was issued in 1908 that, since its first appearance, "I...have had no active dealings with the subject; I have had no part in its important development and I could add nothing fresh to what was written in 1895."[11] The time-consuming nature of the cathartic treatment was simply incompatible with the nature of his general practice, which in any event amply sufficed to secure for him a lucrative living.

For Freud, by contrast, circumstances were quite otherwise. He had already, in his own words,

> abandoned the treatment of organic nervous diseases, but that was of little importance. For on the one hand the prospects in the treatment of such disorders were in any case never promising, while on the other hand, in the private practice of a physician working in a large town, the quantity of such patients was nothing compared to the crowds of neurotics...[12]

In the last half of the 1890s and a for a few years beyond, hysteria continued to be a focus, indeed had come to dominate, both his clinical practice and his intellectual horizons. His thinking on the subject, and his modes of dealing with his patients, had begun to move in very different directions, and had formed the basis for the construction of a new theory of mind, one that extended to encompass the "normal" as well as the pathological. Simultaneously, they constituted the occasion for developing a new technology of treatment.

To argue that hysteria was at root a psychological, not a physical, disorder was a risky move. As Freud would acknowledge in the opening lecture he delivered in America on psychoanalysis in 1909, the doctor does not have the same sympathy for the former as for the latter…all his knowledge—his training in anatomy, in physiology, and in pathology—leaves him in the lurch when he is confronted with hysterical phenomena…So it comes about that hysterical patients forfeit his sympathy. He regards them as people who are transgressing the laws of science—like heretics in the eyes of the orthodox. He attributes every kind of wickedness to them, accuses them of exaggeration, of deliberate deceit, of malingering. And he punishes them by withdrawing his interest from them.[13]

It was an abdication of clinical responsibility that Freud would refuse, and an intellectual stance he would repudiate. For him, human psychology was as rule-governed, as deterministic, as the functioning of the human organism, and therefore it followed that to explain hysteria along psychological lines was not in any way to imply that the disorder was under the volitional control of those who suffered from it. Talk of malingering, of deception, of manipulation came only from people "unaccustomed to reckoning with a strict and universal application of determinism to mental life."[14]

In 1896, the year after *Studies in Hysteria* had appeared in print, Freud published three papers outlining a theory that traced the disease to a different sort of repressed memory, a remembrance of sexual seduction or abuse in infancy. Breuer had recognized that there was frequently a sexual component in cases of hysteria. Freud, however, was now asserting something much stronger: that sexual trauma was always and everywhere the root cause of the disorder. Here was "the key that unlocks everything."[15] If reflex theories had linked hysteria to female reproductive organs, Freud's psychological theories now traced it back to repressed memories of sexual molestation and incestuous assaults as a child. Sex and psychopathology remained inextricably bound up with each other, but now in novel forms.

Even the prominent Viennese sexologist Richard von Krafft-Ebbing, recently installed in Meynert's chair at the University of Vienna and the most powerful psychiatrist in Vienna, thought this a bit much, openly dismissing Freud's theory as "a scientific fairy-tale."[16] And, within a year, Freud was off on another tack: the repressed "memories" of childhood seduction were fantasies, not real events. The florid bodily symptoms of his hysterical patients were the somatic conversions of psychological distress, and reading those symptoms, exploring their roots, required the construction of a whole new theory of the human mind. It was an exploratory trip in which hypnosis was of very little use. Instead, the patient's free associations, alongside dreams and slips of the tongue, were to provide, in the hands of Freud and his followers, a new guide to the complexity of the territory.

Only a handful of people have followed the renegade Freudian analyst and Sanskrit scholar Jeffrey Moussaieff Masson in seeing Freud's abandonment of seduction theory as a form of intellectual cowardice or bad faith. For most, whether drawn from the dwindling ranks of the Freudian true believers or from those who regard psychoanalysis as an interesting and curious, if dated and superseded, historical phenomenon, Freud's own reasons for discarding his belief in the literal truth of most accounts of childhood sexual abuse have been seen as plausible. His treatments based on this theory had almost universally failed, and he had discovered no sure way to distinguish between memories of "real" abuse and fantasies. If that were not bad enough, the sheer number of hysterics flocking to him for treatment seemed to imply that, if hysteria was the product of prior assault, an extraordinarily high number of fathers were pedophiles, a claim he found increasingly implausible. Adding to his discomfort on the latter score was the fact that he himself had suffered from a hysterical breakdown in the late 1990s, following the death of his father on October 23, 1896. He was depressed, riven with self-doubts, and obsessively preoccupied with thoughts of his own premature death; he experienced regular gastric upsets and convinced himself that he was suffering from cardiac problems. Some of his siblings also manifested hysterical symptoms. Did that mean that his father was a child abuser? That, for Freud, was going too far. Instead, by analyzing himself and his dreams, and setting those experiences alongside what he learned from other patients, he moved towards a wholly psychological account of the origins of hysteria.

It was an account that placed fantasy at the root of neurosis, and elaborated a complex model of just how aspects of child development that were supposed to correspond to a universal human nature might under certain conditions provoke hysteria and other forms of psychopathology. That model took a decade and more to develop (and would continue to be modified and tweaked thereafter), but, with the publication of *Three Essays on the Theory of Sexuality* in 1905, its central elements became clear. The central psychological underpinning for all humans was the libido, the energy that was supplied by unconscious sexual drives. "It is the sexual function," he announced, "that I look upon as the foundation of hysteria and of the psychoneuroses in general."[17] All sorts of psychological conflicts and discomforts flowed from that fundamental reality.

The Freudian unconscious was a fearful place, one made and generally marred from the outset by the looming presence of parental figures in the newborn's mental universe. So, far from being a haven from a heartless world, the family was the arena for a host of frightful and dangerous psychodramas that populated that unconscious, fomented its repressions, and created its psychopathologies. As the infant struggled to grow up, and the child to mature, the perils of Oedipal conflicts awaited, and too often wreaked havoc. Forced to repress unacceptable desires, and to deny their fantasies, or to drive them underground, children were riven with psychical conflict. Cravings and suppressions, a search for substitute satisfactions, false forgetting, the constraints of "civilized" morality—in all these respects and more the conflict between Eros and Psyche created a minefield from which few emerged unscathed and unscarred.

If hysteria became just one among many forms of psychopathology Freud and his growing band of followers sought to explain and treat, it nonetheless deserves much of the credit (or blame) for the birth of psychoanalysis, a set of doctrines and practices that would prove of growing significance in the twentieth century—indeed, one that would come to dominate American psychiatry for a quarter of a century and more in the years immediately following the Second World War. And yet the ranks of the classic hysterics, both the sorts of patients Freud had observed at the Salpêtrière, and those he and Breuer had jointly written about, mysteriously seemed to thin out by the end of the nineteenth century, or soon thereafter. One more famous hysterical patient came Freud's way, however, in October 1900, at a time when clients were particularly thin on the ground: Ida Bauer, a woman known to posterity as "Dora." Dora's case would allow Freud to incorporate dream analysis into his discussion of hysteria, and it would prompt him to write still another novelistic case history of a young woman afflicted with a protean array of symptoms, the *Fragment of a Case of Hysteria*.

Dora arrived on Freud's doorstep at her father's insistence. The perversity of that action would become fully apparent only as the case unfolded, and would almost be matched, one might conclude, by the nature of the treatment and the interpretations of her "illness" that Freud sought to provide. Ostensibly, the 17-year-old Dora's encounter with Freud was provoked by her parents' discovery of a suicide note in her room. That gesture followed two years of depression and difficulty eating, and repeated quarrels with both her mother and her father. On one occasion, these had provoked convulsions and a fainting fit, about which she professed to be amnesiac. Over a period lasting several years, from the age of 13, she had spoken of fatigue and difficulties in concentrating, and her social contacts had steadily diminished. Even before these symptoms surfaced, she had suffered from migraines, had developed a persistent cough, and had periodically lost her voice. Electrotherapy and hydrotherapy had been tried, but with little success.

"Dora's" father, Philipp Bauer, was already on friendly terms with Freud, who had treated him in years past for tertiary syphilis, so his referral of his daughter for treatment of her "hysterical" symptoms was apparently unsurprising. But once Freud began his "talking cure" a rather more sinister story began to emerge. A prosperous textile manufacturer, Philipp had moved to Meran (now Merano) in the Alps as part of his treatment for tuberculosis. Here, he and his wife became acquainted with the K.'s, a younger family residing in the neighborhood. When syphilis complicated his tuberculosis, Frau K. became his nurse. Soon, the two were lovers, and Frau K. broke off sexual relations with her husband. In turn, Herr K. began to pay close attention to young Dora. One day, he arranged to meet her (together with his wife) at a church. Dora arrived to find he was alone. He drew the shutters

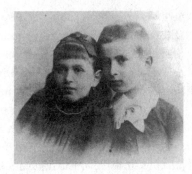

17. "Dora" (Ida Bauer) (1882–1945) with her brother Otto, aged 8 and 9 respectively. Her presentation as a sexual prize to Herr K., and her subsequent encounter with Freud, were still a few years away. (*Verein für Geschichte der Arbeiterbewegung*)

on the windows, pulled her to him, and attempted to kiss her. She responded by slapping him and running away. Two summers later, when she was 15, Herr K. renewed his attentions, propositioning her sexually, and remarking "You know I get nothing out of my wife." Again, she ran from the scene. That afternoon, waking from a nap, she found Herr K. standing at her bedside. When she informed her mother and then her father of these episodes, she was treated as though she were delusionary. Repeatedly, she begged her father to break off relations with the K.'s, only to be ignored, till the truth finally dawned on her: "she had been handed over to Herr K. as the price for his tolerating the relations between her father and his wife."[18] Hence her unremitting depression.

Such, however, was not Freud's interpretation of her problems. Relentlessly, he pressed upon the abused adolescent an alternative view of her sufferings. Her disgust at Herr K.'s attempted kiss disguised the fact that she really wanted to be kissed. Her reaction, when surely she secretly welcomed such advances, reflected her repression of her real wishes, and signaled that she was "entirely and completely hysterical." A dream she reported of her father rescuing her from a burning house, the same house where Herr K. had tried to seduce her, was in reality a disguised acknowledgment of the flames of sexual desire, while other aspects of the dream showed that she masturbated, and had fantasies of oral sex with her father. As evidence, he pointed to her nervous habit of playing with her purse, opening it, sticking a finger into it, and then closing it. Surely the symbolic significance of what she was up to was obvious. And so forth. Repeatedly, Freud invoked his authority as her therapist in an attempt to browbeat an anguished adolescent whose father had offered her up as a sexual prize to the middle-aged man he was cuckolding.

Three months after she had reluctantly undertaken treatment with Freud, Dora abruptly broke off her analysis in anger and disgust, and flounced out of his consulting rooms. Who can blame her? In Erik Erikson's words, "Dora had been traumatized, and Freud retraumatized her." Her treatment at his hands, Erikson concluded, "is one of the great psychotherapeutic disasters; one of the most remarkable exhibitions of a clinician's published rejection of his patient; spectacular, though tragic, evidence of sexual abuse of a young girl, and her own analyst's exoneration of that abuse; an eminent case of forced associations, forced remembering, and perhaps several forced dreams."[19] As a parting shot, when he published the case, Freud suggested that she harbored bisexual longings towards Frau K., the remaining adult in her circle, to whom Dora had turned in her distress.

Perhaps Dora should have been grateful, though. At least she was not seduced by her therapist (though Freud had suggested to her, on the basis of still another of her dreams, that she must want to kiss him, since he was an avid smoker, like both her father and Herr K.). From Ernest Jones fleeing London in the wake of sexual scandal and allegations of child abuse, through Jung's seduction of the disturbed Sabina Spielrein (not the last of his predatory affairs with patients), and Sándor Ferenczi's affair with both Gizella Pallos and her daughter Elma (both of whom had been his analysands), not to mention the wilder escapades of such people as Wilhelm Reich and Otto Gross, the roll of sexual dishonor among psychoanalysts is long. The joining of sex, hysteria, and psychoanalysis occurred, it would seem, on many levels.

Dora's departure from Freud's couch broadly coincided with a shift in the focus of much of his clinical activity toward other forms of neurosis. More generally, the sorts of dramatic somatization that were so notable a feature of the *fin-de-siècle* landscape seem somehow to have disappeared, or at least vanished from view. When hysteria once more appeared in dramatic guise on the historical stage, its victims would be men, not women, and they would number in the tens of thousands, perhaps even the hundreds of thousands. These psychically wounded souls would remain anonymous for the most part, not the individualized, identifiable cases of a Freud or a Charcot. But much of their suffering, too, would come to be viewed through a psychological lens. Sometimes that interpretation would allow a certain sympathy for their condition. More often, it would provoke the veiled hostility and sadism toward them that had characterized many previous medical responses to hysteria. For what could be more unmanly and contemptible than a male hysteric?

VIII

THE WOUNDS OF WAR

We dredged him up, for killed, until he whined
"Oh sir, my eyes—I'm blind,—I'm blind, I'm blind!"
Coaxing, I held a flame against his lids
And said if he could see the least blurred light
He was not blind; in time he'd get it right.
"I can't," he sobbed.

            …one sprang up, and stared
With piteous recognition in fixed eyes,
Lifting distressful hands, as if to bless.
And by his smile, I knew that sullen hall,—
By his dead smile I knew we stood in Hell.

                          Wilfred Owen

They'll soon forget their haunted nights; their cowed
    Subjection to the ghosts of friends who died,—
Their dreams that drip with murder; and they'll be proud
    Of glorious war that shatter'd all their pride…
    Men who went out to battle, grim and glad;
    Children, with eyes that hate you, broken and mad.

                        Siegfried Sassoon

On August 14, 1914, the war to end all wars began. It was destined to be, in the words of the eminent German sociologist Max Weber, a "great and wonderful war."[1] Civilization (whichever version of civilization one's side was defending) would triumph, and the barbarians on the other side would be decisively defeated. And it would all be over by Christmas. Perhaps sooner: the Kaiser, seeing his troops off to the front in the first week of August, informed them: "You will be home before the leaves have fallen from the trees."[2]

Except that they weren't. Far from it. Instead, the conflict would drag on and on, and then drag on some more, on its Western Front chewing up the landscape of northern and eastern France, and, even more dramatically, chewing up a whole generation of young men sent off to fight for King and Country, *Kaiser und Reich, Président et patrie, Donaumonarch und Kaisertum Österreich.* Amidst the mud and the muck of the fields of Flanders, through the valley of the Somme, and all the way down to the Swiss border, millions of brave men would perish, and for what few afterwards could say. But alongside the corpses and those mutilated in body, a new kind of casualty of the killing fields soon began to surface, to infuriate the generals, to threaten morale and the ability to fight, and to occupy the attentions of the medical men charged with coping with battlefield casualties: the victims of what Charles Myers, a Cambridge medic and psychologist turned army doctor, famously called "shell shock."

It was a condition that, for the careful observer, had been foreshadowed in the Boer War at the turn of the century and in the Balkan War of 1912–13, even among some of the survivors of America's great bloodletting, the Civil War, many of whom had flocked to the neurologists' consulting rooms in its aftermath.

But psychiatric misfits materialized in 1914 and 1915 on a scale and in dramatic forms that made them impossible to ignore. And in the remaining years of the war and its immediate aftermath, shell shock became epidemic, even as the military brass forbade the use of the term. "War," in Sir Michael Howard's apt phrase, "was a test of manhood"[3]—and it was a test, under the new conditions of industrialized warfare, that many seemed destined to fail. Were such men mad, or merely malingering, sick, or slyly evading their duty?

The first months of the war brought a rapid German advance, and then stalemate and bloodshed on a massive scale, sufficient, for example, essentially to wipe out the pre-war professional British army by December 1914. But a legion of patriotic volunteers hastened to replace their ranks, and the war machine relentlessly ground on. By 1916 the British found they had to institute conscription; the French had seen near mutiny among their troops (and almost half their army would mutiny in the spring of 1917); and the Germans and the Austrians had lost any illusions about the brevity of the war but clung to a determination "to see it through." Dug into an elaborate series of trenches protected by barbed wire, the opposing armies faced each other across no-man's-land, periodically launching suicidal assaults that moved the front a few hundred yards east or west, and then losing the territory bought with so much blood not long afterwards. Nowhere was this cycle to be more evident than in the terrible series of battles in 1917 near Ypres, known to the British as Passchendaele. Here, where the water table lay too close to the surface to permit proper trenching, the assaults proved particularly murderous. During one battle, amidst torrential downpours, the soldiers crawled into shell holes created by the thousands of rounds of artillery launched by both sides, seeking some margin of safety. During the night, one junior officer, Edwin Vaughan, lay and listened.

> From other shell holes from the darkness on all sides came the groans and wails of wounded men; faint, long sobbing moans of agony, and despairing shrieks. It was too horribly obvious that dozens of men with serious wounds must have crawled for safety into new shell holes, and now the water was rising about them and, powerless to move, they were slowly drowning. Horrible visions came to me with those cries, [of men] lying maimed out there trusting that their pals would find them, and now dying terribly, alone amongst the dead in the inky darkness. And we could do nothing to help them…[By morning] the cries of the wounded had much diminished…and as we staggered down the road, the reason was only too apparent, for the water was right over the tops of the shell holes.[4]

By the end of 1917, a million French soldiers had been killed, out of a male population of perhaps twenty million, 640,000 of them in the first year and a half of the war. German casualties were even higher, because they were fighting on two fronts: a million of their troops had been killed by the end of 1916. The British lost 90,000 men by November 1914. At the Somme offensive, which began on July 1, 1916, 20,000 British troops were killed and 40,000 were wounded on the first day alone, slaughtered by German machine guns and artillery as they marched futilely forward, never, in most instances, even reaching the German trenches. Many of the wounded died agonizing drawn-out deaths where they lay over the next several days, beyond the reach of rescue. By month's end, the English and French had lost 200,000 men, and the Germans 160,000, and the industrialized killing had moved the front barely 3 miles. When the "offensive" was officially abandoned on November 19, stopped by the rising tide of mud, each side had suffered over 600,000 casualties.

But it was not just the pointless sacrifice, the mass slaughter, and the sight of the maimed and frightfully wounded that wore on men's nerves. Almost worse was the daily sense of fear and loss of control, and the tension caused by the inability to escape from an intolerable situation. All the while, of course, officers and men were meant to obey the injunction to display unnatural courage, even when a high-explosive projectile might, at any instant and without any warning, end one's existence. Both "must remain for days, weeks, even months, in a narrow trench or stuffy dugout, exposed to constant danger of the most fearful kind; namely, bombardment with high explosive shells, which comes from some unseen source, and against which no personal agility or wit is of any avail."[5] That was the existential reality of a war of attrition, conducted with high explosives, with flesh-tearing weapons (bullets, bayonets), and ultimately even with the horrors of poison gas, by politicians and generals seemingly—and all too often actually—without conscience.

Perhaps it should occasion no surprise that, under such circumstances, many officers and enlisted men proved unequal to the task. No army was spared the epidemic of nervous disease that seemed to strike at an accelerating pace. The effects on military preparedness and military morale threatened to become overwhelming. What was one to make of soldiers who suddenly lost the power of speech or hearing; who professed to be blind; who stammered, or twisted convulsively, or walked with a peculiar and unnatural gait; who wept or screamed unceasingly, or displayed other symptoms of uncontrollable emotionality; who claimed their limbs were paralyzed; who claimed to have lost all memory; who could not sleep, or who, if sleeping, experienced the most frightful nightmares that left them bereft of rest and on the verge of collapse; who suddenly, in other words, manifested physical symptoms that rendered the notion of sending them into battle apparently absurd?

For many of the military brass, the answer was obvious: these creatures were unmanly cowards and malingerers, seeking to shirk their patriotic duty. They should be offered the choice of abandoning their "pretended" illnesses, or being shot. A relative handful did suffer the latter fate, but ordering firing squads to kill, not just a dozen or two of their comrades, but thousands and even tens of thousands of them, was perhaps too much even for the generals (and if not for them, certainly too much for the civilians behind the lines to stomach). Army medics were perforce handed a dual task: to explain what had gone wrong; and to develop remedies that would, in the shortest time possible and to the maximum extent possible, return those they treated to the military machine so that they could kill and be killed.

The term "shell shock" encapsulates one initially plausible account of the mass breakdowns. The concussive force of the high-explosive projectiles that rained down on the troops traumatized the bodies of those exposed to it. Shells that exploded were a novel form of weaponry, and many thought that the blast that accompanied their arrival inflicted invisible injuries to the bodies of those exposed to the explosion, even those who initially appeared unharmed. Their nervous systems were damaged in subtle if not directly observable ways: tears to the spinal cord, or minute hemorrhages and micropunctures of the brain. Some even speculated that winds generated by passing machine gun bullets mimicked the effects of shell blast, or that the problems were caused by the poison gases released by the explosions. It was these real, but undetectable, bodily injuries that were the cause of the soldiers' symptoms.

Such theories had the distinct advantage of providing the sort of somatic etiology that doctors preferred, but, given that the postulated traumatic injuries were undemonstrable, they had the equally distinct *dis*advantage of encouraging malingerers to simulate the behaviors that provoked the diagnosis, potentially a disaster for the military machine. Besides, accumulating evidence cast doubt on the premise: soldiers who had never been within miles of the front exhibited the signs of shell shock; the physically injured and maimed likewise seemed remarkably exempt from its ravages; prisoners of war, safe from further physical danger, were miraculously spared the symptoms. Some neurologists and army medics found ways to sustain their belief in "shock" as a genuine cause of the cases that came before them. Many more, however, saw stress and suggestibility as the root of the evil.

Even in these cases, however, ways of framing mental disease that pre-dated the war offered the intellectual resources to rescue a physical account of the disorders. The degenerationist theories that had dominated asylum medicine from the last third of the nineteenth century forwards had already been employed by Charcot to "explain" hysteria. Many were drawn to a similar account of shell shock. It had, these doctors acknowledged, a psychological component, as the cruelties and pressures of trench warfare relentlessly wore upon the men. But, in the words of one of Britain's leading alienists, Charles Mercier, mental disorder did not occur in "people who are of sound mental constitution. It does not, like smallpox and malaria, attack indifferently the weak and the strong. It occurs chiefly in those whose mental constitution is originally defective, and whose defect is manifested in the lack of the power of self-control and of forgoing immediate indulgence."[6] Such degenerates were almost as defective physically as mentally—weak, terrified, and decrepit souls whose breakdowns were thoroughly predictable and had little to do with the exigencies of war; or else cowardly malingerers shirking their duty to comrades, king, and country—people deserving harsh treatment rather than sympathy and pensions.

Similar ideas were embraced by many French and German physicians. Charcot's student Josef Babinski, for example (known today mostly for his eponymous reflex), had done much to discredit the work of his *maître* once the grand old man was safely dead. Babinski had insisted that, under Charcot, the boundaries of hysteria had been drawn far too broadly. Most patients had, in reality, been suffering from real neurological illnesses that had simply been misdiagnosed. The small subset of hysterics that remained was suffering from a condition he proposed—as we have previously seen—ought to be renamed *pithiatisme*, which meant "curable by persuasion." If "persuasion" might cure such cases, it was suggestion, he argued, that had provoked them. But only the already defective would have succumbed, since "one must be abnormal to be susceptible to suggestion"[7]—a variant of the idea that only the degenerate were hypnotizable. Before the war, Babinski's ideas were deeply controversial in many quarters, but the epidemic of shell shock brought a reappraisal. If the victims of this syndrome were hysterics, then their symptoms were the product of suggestion, and they might be "persuaded" to abandon them. Quite how that persuasion might be accomplished was, of course, the crucial question.

In the 1880s and 1890s, the courts in Britain, the United States, and Germany had seen a rash of claims from those victimized by accidents in the workplace or in train crashes. As well as those with obvious physical illnesses, there were others who displayed the symptoms of a traumatic neurosis, and a fierce controversy had erupted between those who claimed that "railway spine" and the like were the result of real physical trauma too subtle for existing instruments to detect, and those who saw them as "hysterical" forms of malingering, created by suggestions from complaisant physicians and the prospect of financial compensation. Such debates grew particularly fierce in Bismarck's Germany, where the legislation of 1884 giving pensions to the victims of railway and industrial accidents had been extended in 1889 to cover mental and nervous debility. Critics had charged that the epidemic of "pension neurosis" and insurance fraud was a direct result of the financial incentives this legislation created. No pensions, no pathological and pathogenic delusions and desires, and no neuroses. If the complaints were "mere hysteria," then work, not pension-supported idleness, beckoned—a stance that, as Paul Lerner has argued, created a "uniquely German" impetus to dislodge hysteria "from its exclusive association with women."[8]

Hermann Oppenheim, who had been the most vigorous proponent of the contrary proposition—that these travails were symptomatic of real somatic trauma—remained true to his beliefs when he encountered the first psychiatric casualties of the war. But now his assertions were viewed not just as economically costly, but as dangerous to the war effort, and thus unpatriotic. German psychiatrists hastened to a meeting in Munich in September 1916, at which Oppenheim was ritually humiliated, his claims discredited, his authority as a professional stripped away. Just as his earlier doctrines were alleged to have helped to create "the heavy burden of thousands of work-shy individuals...the accident hysterics, whose epidemic appearance was made possible by the introduction of an intangible and uncontrollable concept"—traumatic neurosis—so a repetition of the error in wartime would, as one German psychiatrist put it, "artificially create an epidemic of war neurosis."[9]

Henceforth, no one of any consequence on the German side of the lines dissented from the notion that "shell shock" was simply male hysteria, a flight into illness to escape hellish dangers. Karl Bonhoeffer, for instance, had treated soldiers from both sides after the battle of Verdun. It was enough to convince him that

> the hysterical reactions are the result of the more or less conscious wish for self-preservation. The difference in behaviour between the Germans who came directly from the line of fire into the hospital station and the French prisoners was striking. Among the Germans the familiar forms of hysterical reactions could be found with great frequency, while among the French, who had come from the same front circumstances, no trace of hysteria was to be seen. For them, the danger had disappeared. "Ma guerre est fini," was the common turn of phrase. There was, hence, no longer any reason for an illness to develop.

No wonder many German psychiatrists came to call shell shock *Shreckneurose*, or "terror neurosis."[10]

If the French and the Germans thus converged on the notion that shell shock was a mass epidemic of male hysteria, many British doctors as well were coming to see shell shock in increasingly psychological terms. Unbearable tension, fear, disgust, grief, horror, a litany of strong emotions and frightful experiences were seen as the possible precipitants of a "flight into illness." To employ an anachronistic term, they recognized that both officers and men were trapped in a double-bind: their powerful drives toward self-preservation could find no obvious outlet. To flee would invite being shot as a deserter, and would for many be a deeply cowardly and "unmanly" act. To stay meant more daily trauma, from which the only possible release seemed to be death. Hence the development of psychosomatic symptoms: mutism, hysterical blindness, uncontrollable shaking, paralyses, disturbances of sleep and gait, disorientation, and cardiac palpitations—so-called soldier's heart. Now an inability to perform one's duty had a "physical" cause.

It did not go unremarked that many of the psychological mechanisms that produced this epidemic of male hysteria could be understood in terms of the intellectual theories of hysteria and neurosis that had been developed by Freud and his followers. The role of traumatic memories, the attempts at repression, the conversion of mental conflicts into physical symptomatology, the significance of dreams, the value of abreaction and catharsis, the very notion that hysteria could be understood and explained in psychological terms: these were all elements of the Freudian corpus that were incorporated into the understanding and to some degree the therapy of shell shock. To be sure, therapeutic interventions along psychotherapeutic lines were largely (and for obvious reasons) confined to the officer class, who, incidentally, suffered from shell shock at four or five times the rate found among enlisted men. And the adoption of a modified psychoanalytic schema was made easier because of the perceived irrelevance of Freud's claims about the etiological significance of childhood and sex to hysteria in shell-shock cases, since these two elements were always the aspect of his theories with which most Edwardian doctors were most uncomfortable. What that meant, of course, as Janet Oppenheim has trenchantly pointed out, was that "Freud's work was, in fact, eviscerated for its first significant application in Great Britain and, no doubt, that operation made it more palatable to a suspicious public, ready to reject 'Teutonic science' out of hand."[11]

If the larger framework that had suggested their relevance had been castrated, to employ a slightly different surgical metaphor, in its reduced state, the Freudian emphasis on dreams, trauma, and mental conflicts undoubtedly drew considerable attention from a number of physicians as the war wore on. The psychiatrist John T. MacCurdy, visiting soldiers under treatment in England in 1917, encountered a young British lieutenant who had fought bravely at the front since the early months of the war. Escalating nightmares and insomnia had led to his breakdown in March. Night after night, he dreamt that "he was back on the Somme front, and being shelled mercilessly. Shells would come closer and closer to him, finally one would land right on top of him and he would awake with a shriek of terror." On other occasions, "when falling off to sleep he would have...hallucinations of Germans entering the room, and with these visions, too, there was great terror." Not surprisingly, "he was in general quite convinced that he was physically and nervously a complete wreck," afraid even to venture out into the hospital grounds.[12] An officer treated in Scotland by the Cambridge physician W. H. R. Rivers had been blown up by an incoming shell and buried by the blast debris, yet somehow survived and continued to fight. Then he went in search of

> a fellow-officer and found his body blown to pieces with head and limbs separated from his trunk...From that time he had been haunted at night by the vision of his dead and mutilated friend. When he slept he had nightmares in which his friend appeared, sometimes as he had seen him mangled

in the field, sometimes in the still more terrifying aspect of one whose limbs and features had been eaten away by leprosy. The mutilated or leprous officer of the dream would come nearer and nearer until the patient suddenly awoke pouring with sweat and in a state of utmost terror.[13]

For others, the nightmares involved no distortion of reality, merely an incessant replaying of the event that had driven them over the edge. Dreams were bad, but memories were often worse. The pre-eminent American brain surgeon Harvey Cushing, then a young army medic, later recalled an equally young "Captain B." telling him:

> The chief trouble now is dreams—not exactly dreams, either, but right in the middle of an ordinary conversation the face of a Boche that I have bayoneted comes sharply into view, or I see the man whose head one of our boys took off with a blow on the back of his neck with a bolo knife, and the blood spurted high in the air before the body fell. And the horrible smells! You know I can hardly see meat come on the table.[14]

Death was omnipresent. Wilhelm Reich recalled "barbed-wire fences, hung with bodies." Battlefields were littered with corpses.

> What good does it do to cover them with sand and lime, or to throw a tent half over them, in order to escape their black, bloated faces? There were too many. Everywhere, shovels struck something buried. All the secrets of the grave lay open in a grotesquerie worse than the most lunatic dream. Hair fell in clumps from skulls like rotting leaves from autumn trees. Some decayed into a green fish-flesh, which gleamed at night through the torn uniforms.[15]

Even worse experiences awaited some poor souls. The use of poison gas by both sides—chlorine and the still more damaging phosgene in 1915, and by 1918 "mustard gas"—led to horrific deaths. Those who donned their primitive masks quickly enough were forced to watch the gruesome effects on their comrades who were not so lucky: lungs filling with liquid that caused slow suffocation; water and blood flowing from the mouths of victims as their internal organs were reduced to slime and collapsed; throats, lungs, and eyes blistered and burned, producing a slow and agonizing death, "white eyes writhing," "blood...gargling from the froth-corrupted lungs."[16] W. H. R. Rivers, who treated shell-shocked officers sent from the front to Craiglockhart in Scotland, encouraged them to speak of their trauma, seeking to produce a catharsis. But one case, in particular, defeated his best efforts. The young man had been

> flung down by the explosion of a shell so that his face struck the abdomen of a German several days dead, the impact of his fall rupturing the swollen corpse. Before he lost consciousness, the patient had clearly realized his situation and knew that the substance which filled his mouth and produced the most horrible sensations of taste and smell was derived from the decomposed entrails of an enemy.[17]

No wonder this patient routinely vomited when called upon to eat.

In 1918 the American artist John Singer Sargent painted the enormous canvass *Gassed*, after being sent to the front to portray the cooperation between British and American troops. At a casualty station near Arras, he saw an orderly leading a group of soldiers blinded by mustard gas. Beyond their devastating direct effects on the unprotected, gas attacks had a deeply traumatic effect on those who survived. Sargent's painting, in choosing to adopt the conventions of the frieze, somewhat undercuts the horrors of such scenes, horrors that are more vividly and memorably captured in the bitter lines of Wilfred Owen's "Dulce et Decorum Est" (1917).

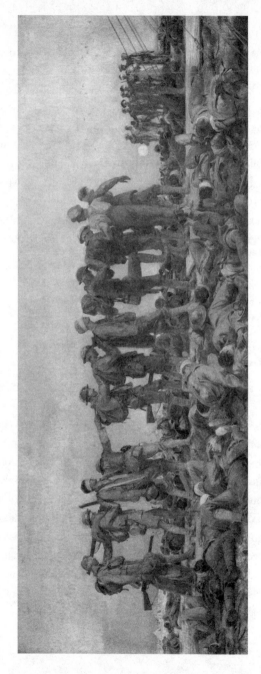

18. *Gassed*, by the American artist John Singer Sargent, an enormous canvass (7½ ft. × 20 ft.) that hangs in the Imperial War Museum in London. (*Imperial War Museum*)

Gas! Gas! Quick, boys! An ecstasy of fumbling,
Fitting the clumsy helmets just in time,
But someone still was yelling out and stumbling
And floundering like a man in fire or lime.
Dim through the misty panes and thick green light,
As under a green sea, I saw him drowning.
In all my dreams, before my helpless sight,
He plunges at me, guttering, choking, drowning.

If in some smothering dreams, you too could pace
Behind the wagon that we flung him in.
And watch the white eyes writing in his face,
His hanging face, like a devil's sick of sin;
If you could hear at every jolt, the blood
Come gargling from the froth-corrupted lungs,
Obscene as cancer, bitter as the cud
Of vile, incurable sores on innocent tongues,
My friend, you would not tell with such high zest
To children ardent for some desperate glory,
The old Lie: Dulce et decorum est,
Pro patria mori.

Thomas Salmon, the American psychiatrist, was another contemporary observer who noted a close correspondence between the hysterical symptoms of patients and their particular wartime experiences: "Thus a soldier who bayonets an enemy in the face develops a hysterical tic of his facial muscles; abdominal contractions occur in men who have bayoneted enemies in the abdomen; hysterical blindness follows particularly horrible sights; hysterical deafness appears in men who find the cries of the wounded unbearable, and the men attached to burial parties develop amnesia."[18] Reality was, of course, never so neat, but for those who made such connections, the psychogenic origins of shell shock were too obvious and powerful to ignore.

Still, even these modified psychoanalytic accounts of this epidemic of male hysteria always remained a minority taste, just as only a comparative handful of shell-shock victims were treated with sympathetic attention, talk therapy, and hypnosis. But, because the men in question were officers, and, in a number of instances, major war poets, whose images of the trenches haunt even the contemporary imagination—men such as Wilfred Owen and Siegfried Sassoon—disproportionate attention has been lavished on them and those who treated them, W. H. R. Rivers, A. J. Brock, and others. They have even materialized in fictional and filmic form—for example, in Pat Barker's *Resurrection* trilogy, and the film derived from the books, *Regeneration* (released in the United States as *Behind the Lines*).

Because the treatment of an Owen or a Sassoon was relatively humane (though ultimately still designed to return them to the killing fields, where Owen would die, ironically after the war's official end), and because of the stark contrast that exists in the treatment of many of the "other ranks," it would be easy to construct a link between the recognition of shell shock's psychogenic origins and a more understanding, "kinder" therapy. Easy, but wrong. Whichever side of the mortal combat one examines, the more common link is between an assimilation of shell shock to the pre-war conceptions of hysteria, and the infliction of painful, almost sadistic, remedies.

Perhaps that should occasion little surprise. After all, however much one insisted that the symptoms were the product of the unconscious, the idea that hysteria was "all in the mind" conjured up uncomfortable echoes of the generals' conviction that it was all fakery and weakness of the will. The line between shell shock and cowardice seemed blurred at best, and many of the doctors who treated hysterical soldiers were only a little less inclined than their military superiors to conflate the two. So far as they could tell, "hysterical" paralyses and the faked paralysis of the malingerer were equally unanchored in any real neurological disorder, and both reflected an enfeeblement of the will. With immense pressures on the medics to return as many patients as possible to the front lines, and little official concern with the long-term psychological state of the cannon fodder, the temptation to resort to autocratic, sometimes brutal, forms of treatment was great.

There were some experiments with hypnotism, notably by the charismatic Max Nonne, who treated some of the German troops, but few could replicate the dramatic results he claimed to obtain. Instead, direct attempts to strengthen the will and to induce the soldier to relinquish his symptoms were far more prevalent. Independently, the French, the Germans, the Austrians, and the British all responded to the catastrophic threat to military manpower by employing a mixture of "conscious suggestion" reinforced by electrotherapy. There were remarkable overlaps in the different approaches. In Germany, a Fritz Kaufmann invented what was quickly dubbed the "Kaufmann cure,"[19] the use of a combination of electricity and forced military drill, to the accompaniment of loudly shouted orders. Intense and painful electrical stimulation was applied to apparently paralyzed limbs for several minutes on a repeated basis, for hours at a time, till the patient gave way and the hysterical paralysis resolved itself. Among the Austrian troops, under the supervision of Julius von Wagner-Jauregg, the Professor of Psychiatry at the University of Vienna, a Dr Kozlowski applied powerful electrical shocks to men's mouths and their testicles, forcing other shell-shocked soldiers to observe the "treatment" they were about to undergo.

The British might (and did) denounce these activities as further evidence of the depravity of the Huns, but only by mobilizing a not-atypical hypocrisy. For they and their French allies employed almost precisely the same weapons on their own men. Babinski, who had insisted from the start that shell shock was simply the product of hysterical suggestion, advocated, in Marc Roudebush's words, "a direct and systematic assault on the psychological defenses of hysterical patients."[20] Other French neurologists hastened to give substance to his recommendations. Along the banks of the Loire, Clovis Vincent set up his re-education camp. Here, *torpillage*, the use of electrodes designed to deliver a fearsomely sharp galvanic current to the patient's body to "encourage" the paralyzed to move, was accompanied by other techniques deliberately designed to frighten the patient. Vincent added the force of his own personality, and an absolutely implacable demeanor to the occasion, insisting that the single treatment would continue as long as necessary to overcome the "debility of self-control and of the will." In the words of André Gilles, an enthusiastic disciple, "these pseudo-impotents of the voice, of the arms or legs, are really only impotents of the will; it is the doctor's job to will on their behalf."[21] Treatment must be swift and merciless.

Lewis Yealland, a young Canadian doctor practicing at the Queen Square Neurological Hospital in London, and his colleague Edgar Adrian (later to win a Nobel Prize) agreed completely. Shell shock developed "as a result of autosuggestion acting on a mind enfeebled by fear and emotional tension and this autosuggestion becomes so strong that the patient resists all attempts to undermine his fixed belief." In treatment, "he is not asked whether he can raise his paralysed arm or not; he is ordered to raise it and told that he can do it perfectly if he tries.

Rapidity and an authoritative manner are the chief factors in the re-education process." Once again, in case an authoritative command did not suffice, another weapon was held in reserve. A mute soldier is brought into a darkened room, fastened to a chair, and told he must speak. Silence. Mouth propped open with a tongue depressor. A strong electrical current applied to the pharynx. The pain is so excruciating that the soldier arcs back in his chair, tearing the electrodes loose from the battery. Again, they are applied to his throat and he is ordered to speak. After an hour, a muffled "ah." Yealland informs the man that he can and will talk, and will not leave until he does. Hours pass. The man begins to stammer and cry. Not enough. More "strong faradic shocks are applied." The soldier at length talks. Only when he says "thank you" for his cure is he allowed to leave.[22]

For some feminist theorists, the passivity, the impotence, the close confinement of the troops in both the physical and the social sense, their absolute lack of autonomy, their role imprisonment within the confines of the ideology of masculinity and the cult of manliness, and the supposed connections of these constraints to the conversion of their distress into physical symptoms were analogous to the role imprisonment suffered by upper-middle-class Victorian ladies, and the soldiers' hysteria thus directly comparable to theirs. Elaine Showalter has even suggested a further analogy between the brutality of the "therapies" visited upon the shell-shocked, and the sadistic responses of a Brudenell Carter, a Baker Brown, or a Robert Battey to their female hysterical patients. The parallels are interesting on some levels, if easy to overdraw. One wonders, for instance, about how valid it is to compare the wretchedness and brutality of the trenches, the immediate and unceasing threat to the integrity of one's body, indeed one's very existence, to the gilded cage within which a class of privileged women lived—however existentially empty and male-dominated much of their existence proved to be. More seriously, however, such analogies rest on the notion that hysteria was the peculiar province of the female upper classes, a claim that would have astonished Charcot's legions of working-class hysterics, male and female alike, to say nothing of the great man himself. Still, if anyone had doubted the existence of hysteria in the male, the sight of the returning victims of shell shock rudely disposed of that prejudice.

Not that these particular war veterans generally received a warm welcome. The victorious British reneged as often as possible on promises to provide pensions, let alone efforts at treatment, for those who remained battered in mind. In the chaos of a defeated and dismembered Austria–Hungary, as in the struggling post-war Germany, such pathetic figures were a reminder of a bitter defeat, and an impossible drain on a faltering public treasury. The French, as Marc Roudebush has shown, dismissed shell-shocked soldiers as an embarrassment or, worse, a threat to the health and virility of the nation: no pensions or official recognition of their service for them. Only in the United States, perhaps because it had entered the war so late, and so had fewer casualties, or perhaps because of the lobbying efforts of the American Legion, were the shell-shocked veterans eventually accepted as battle-scarred heroes, worthy of acknowledgment and thanks. But then, from its Civil War onwards, the United States has routinely treated its military veterans as the only group worthy of the protections of a welfare state: medical care at public expense; pensions for disabilities; public support for getting an education; and so forth.

As for their doctors, as is customary, those on the winning side escaped all censure. Briefly, it appeared that those on the losing end might be called to account. Their techniques were bitterly resented by the troops and their families, and, in the short revolutionary fever that seized Germany after the Armistice, neurologists were chased from their offices, and there was dark talk of revenge. But the re-establishment of order under the Weimar Republic soon brought such mutterings to naught, and the old hierarchies re-established themselves. In dismembered Austria–Hungary, Wagner-Jauregg found himself on trial for war crimes, the details of his tortures put on public display, only for professional solidarity to trump evidence once more, and for an acquittal to be rendered on all charges. (Wagner-Jauregg would win a Nobel Prize in 1927 for introducing malaria therapy for the treatment of General Paralysis of the Insane, aka tertiary syphilis.) And, with shell shock retreating from public view, the doctors who had sought to treat it largely lost interest, and returned to their peacetime pursuits. The epidemic of male hysteria was no more.

IX

L'HYSTÉRIE MORTE?

Diseases disappear. Occasionally they vanish when public-health campaigns succeed in eliminating all existing outbreaks, and the pathogen responsible for the illness needs a human reservoir and vector to survive. Such was the case with smallpox, whose last remaining case was documented in 1977, and whose demise was announced by the World Health Organization in May 1980. Only the survival of the virus in biological warfare laboratories gives us reason to be concerned about the possible reappearance of an illness that once disfigured and killed on a massive scale. Perhaps polio may soon follow, for new cases of the disease now number in the low hundreds each year, compared with the ten million cases reported as recently as 1988. Occasionally, the discovery of a medical magic bullet ushers a dread disease off the stage. In the early twentieth century, between 15 and 20 per cent of male admissions to New York State's mental hospitals suffered from the ravages of general paresis. In its early stages, the disorder was visible only through subtle signs, overlooked by all but the trained eye—minor disturbances of gait and articulation, the unequal reaction of the pupils to light. But, as the disease unfolded, neurological catastrophes accompanied ever more florid psychiatric symptomatology—delusions of immense sexual prowess, physical strength, wealth, and social power coexisting pathetically in bodies exhibiting progressive paralysis and decay—till fatuity and a dreadful end, flesh rotting and vanishing, bedsores suppurating, mental darkness descending, muscles failing, and death supervening, often from choking on one's own vomit. The discovery that the source of these troubles was the ravages of tertiary syphilis was followed, albeit some decades later, by the introduction of penicillin and other antibiotics, a development that rendered such spectacles moot. No more paretics.

More frequently, though, diseases vanish because medical fashions change, understandings of disease alter, and previous ways of classifying nature and its pathologies are superseded. Where are the dropsies and the relapsing fevers with which every doctor was once familiar? Where are the episodes of chlorosis, or the sthenic and asthenic diseases that loomed so large in nineteenth-century medicine? Gone or reconceptualized every one. More to the point, for our present purposes, where are all the cases of hysteria that once thronged the waiting rooms of the nerve doctors—the paralyses and tics, the phobias and the phantasms, the amnesia and the somnambulism, the hemianesthesia and the histrionics, the inexplicable loss of voice and sight, the emotional turmoil and the faints, and the dramatic muscular contractions that used to culminate in the *arc-en-cercle* so familiar from the beginning to the end of the nineteenth century? Where are the hysterical invalids, so many of them women, who were so visible then?

All apparently vanished into the ether. The new Bible of neo-Kraepelinian mainstream psychiatry, the fourth edition of the *Diagnostic and Statistical Manual* produced by the American Psychiatric Association, can find no place in its vast and ever-expanding array of possible pathologies for a disorder that was once the bread and butter of out-patient neuro-psychiatry, and the inspiration for the theory and practice of Freudian psycho-analysis. Nearly 900 pages and counting, an array of psychiatric disorders now numbering several hundred, and yet no place any longer for hysteria. The term survives in the language, of course, employed as a term of abuse, an epithet most often directed at women who make a spectacle of their extreme emo-tional lability, or invoked when some collective disturbance is dismissed as mass hysteria. But clinicians report that the con-dition itself has shuffled off into oblivion. They have no more hysterics to present at grand rounds, to provide entertainment and enlightenment for their trainees. The disorder that haunted the imagination of the previous *fin de siècle*, the spectacle of the hysterical female (soon joined by legions of male psychiatric casualties of the "war to end all wars"), has apparently evapor-ated. In the words of one of its best-known modern historians, Étienne Trillat, "L'hystérie est morte, c'est entendu."[1]

Its death (if dead it is) was certainly a lingering one. Psychoanalysis, as Carroll Smith-Rosenberg aptly put it, was "the child of the hysterical woman."[2] And parent and child each supported the other, till the collapse of psychoanalysis almost simultaneously brought about the demise of her hysterical par-ent (though in fact hysteria had shown signs of serious decline for some time, and psychoanalysis had long neglected the dis-ease that had brought it into existence).

Freud had stitched together psychoanalysis, as both the-ory and practice, on the foundation of his own hysterical breakdown, and the experience of ministering to a handful of hysterical women in the 1890s. But once he had developed his analytic technique, and constructed his basic model of the conversion of psychic conflicts into physical symptoms, he seems rapidly to have lost interest in the subject. As his intellectual edifice grew ever more complex, and his gaze shifted to the contemplation of the epic problems posed by civilization and its discontents, hysteria quickly lost its initial centrality. Following their master's lead, in this as in all else, Freud's disciples likewise directed their attentions elsewhere. To be sure, those hysterics who showed up to have their psyches rearranged were rarely turned away. They were too lucrative for that. But they seem to have appeared less and less frequently. If psychoanalysts were abandoning hysterics, hysterics also seem to have been deserting psychoanalytic couches in droves.

Most hysterics, it turned out, did not want to be told that their disorders were all in their minds. Victims of a disorder that mysteriously mimicked all sorts of neurological diseases without any obvious organic cause, they were insistent that their disease was a real, physical entity. They did not take kindly to theories that suggested otherwise. It was not just the General Staffs of the First World War armies who equated psychological troubles with malingering and bad faith. Many of the alleged victims of psychopathology shared that view, and loudly proclaimed their entitlement to the status of being genuinely sick. Like the renegade psychiatrist Thomas Szasz, they saw *mental* illness as a fiction and a myth, a term that disparaged the reality of their sufferings and rendered them essentially fraudulent. Besides, the penetration of psychoanalytic ideas and institutions was slow, halting, and uneven. The French, for nationalistic reasons, would have nothing to do with such Teutonic and Semitic doctrines till as late as the 1960s, when they finally emerged in the Frenchified form propounded by Jacques Lacan. In the German-speaking world, the advent of the Nazis soon put paid to Freud's "degenerate" Jewish ideas. And in Britain, with its eclectic psychiatric profession, and its distaste for wallowing in "morbid" introspection, Freudian ideas were never more than a minority taste, mostly confined to the chattering classes, a reality that remained even when Sigmund and Anna Freud were driven into exile in London. To be sure, analytic ideas created a small institutional bridgehead centered around the Tavistock Clinic in London. But the machinations of Edward Mapother and the members of the Institute of Psychiatry ensured that the gates to academic respectability, in the form of an affiliation with the University of London, were firmly shut in the analysts' faces. And the British tradition of emotional reserve kept most affluent patients at bay. Only in the United States, irony of ironies, did psychoanalysis flourish. Freud's contempt for the culture notwithstanding, psychoanalysis attracted a small but growing band of American adherents, professionals and patients, in the years leading up to the war against Hitler and Hirohito, and for a quarter century and more after its end Freudian doctrines became the hegemonic ideology of the American psychiatric elite.

The Second World War, of course, played a major role in the emergence of this dominance. Exploiting the memories of the shell-shocked soldiers of the First World War, American psychiatrists persuaded the military to allow them to examine their recruits to screen out the psychiatrically vulnerable, and so they did, to the tune of nearly two million men rejected as mentally unstable. But it made no difference. Once exposed to the horrors of modern warfare, or sometimes even the prospect of the horrors of the battlefield, the men of "the greatest generation" broke down in large numbers, just as their fathers had before them. There were more than a million admissions to American hospitals in the war years for neuro-psychiatric problems. Among combat units in the European theatre in 1944, admissions were as high as 250 per 1,000 men per year, an extraordinary percentage. "Of the casualties severe enough to require evacuation during the major US campaign in the Pacific, at Guadalcanal in summer and fall 1942, 40 percent were psychiatric."[3] And the surge in the ranks of the psychiatrically impaired showed no signs of diminishing in the immediate aftermath of the conflict. In 1945, 50,662 neuro-psychiatric casualties crowded the wards of military hospitals, and to those who were institutionalized we must add the 475,397 discharged servicemen who were receiving Veterans' Administration pensions for psychiatric disabilities by 1947.

These wartime experiences had a profoundly transformative effect on psychiatry itself. In 1940 psychiatrists had composed a marginal and despised specialty, mostly still trapped within the walls of custodial asylums. The American Psychiatric Association had a total of only 2,295 members. By 1945 the military alone had some 2,400 physicians assigned to psychiatric duties. Many of these doctors had, of course, no prior background in the field, and had been rapidly indoctrinated with a thin veneer of knowledge to allow them to play their expected roles. Nonetheless, they rapidly acquired extensive experience with psychiatric disability, and many of them sought to stay in the field after the war.

The massive number of breakdowns among presumably previously mentally sound soldiers helped to reinforce putative links between overwhelming stress and mental pathology, and, under their psychoanalytically inclined leader, Brigadier

William Menninger, the shock troops of this new wave of psychiatrists readily bought into a psychodynamic account of what was wrong with the soldiers they were charged with treating. Second World War veterans did not have shell shock, but "war neurosis" or "combat exhaustion" proliferated apace. The change in terminology was no accident. The doctors discovered that the less "psychiatric" the diagnosis the better, since a psychiatric label seemed to confirm victims in the sick role and make their recovery unlikely. Better to speak of exhaustion and hustle them back to the fight just as soon as possible. Forward, brief, simplified treatment communicated clearly to patients, treatment personnel, and the combat reference group that psychiatric casualties were unable to function and fight only temporarily. Conversely, evacuation of psychiatric casualties to distant medical facilities "weakened relationships with the combat group and implied failure in battle for which a continuation in the sick role was the only honorable explanation."[4] Giving the soldier a psychiatric diagnosis made that move on the patient's part the more likely, which was why "combat exhaustion" became the preferred term, with its implication that the overtaxed system would recover with little more than a brief rest and respite from the fighting. If a mere psychiatric label had such negative effects on outcomes, sustained psychiatric treatment appeared to make matters even worse, greatly increasing the chances of permanent disability. Whereas there had been debates and then an emerging consensus among many doctors during the First World War that shell shock was a form of masculine hysteria, there were few comparable moves when the next worldwide military conflict exploded.

Three sorts of treatment regime emerged under the pressure to deal with the profound renewed threats to morale and military efficiency that "combat exhaustion" posed: brief interventions lasting a day or two as close to the front lines as possible; removal to a more formal psychiatric facility containing a few hundred beds further up the supply chain, where up to two weeks of more sophisticated treatment were offered; or removal from the battlefield entirely to something that more closely approximated a more traditional mental hospital, where more elaborate interventions could be attempted. The last two venues restored only a very small fraction to a combat role, and many patients treated in them became permanent invalids. And treatment at the front lines generally consisted of little more than warm food and a sedative to secure a good night's sleep, and the mobilization of guilt by the soldiers' doctors, manipulating the soldiers' feelings of solidarity with their units and their desire not to let down their fellow fighting men: an American version of tea and (not too much) sympathy.

On this foundation, American psychiatry in the post-war era swung decisively in a psychoanalytic direction, and it became increasingly an out-patient specialty dealing with the walking wounded. Where virtually the entire membership of the American Psychiatric Association worked in mental hospitals at the end of the 1930s, by 1958 as few as 16 per cent of a greatly expanded profession did so. All those psychiatrists whose livelihood now depended upon an office-based practice naturally gravitated away from the psychotic and towards an ever closer embrace of the various milder "neuroses." It would be natural to conclude, therefore, that hysteria would enjoy a new day in the sun, an expanded place in the theorizing and therapies of the profession. Surely the psychoanalysts now seemingly so securely established as the elite of the American psychiatric profession would renew the focus on a disorder that had given birth to their specialty?

But hysteria turned out to be an elusive quarry. Many of the sufferers had fled, implicitly sharing the biew of turn-of-the-century neurologist J. A. Ormerod that the label had acquired "the disagreeable connotation of a certain moral feebleness in the patient, and of unreality in the symptoms." The Washington psychoanalyst Paul Chodoff commented in 1954 that "hysterical conversion phenomena undoubtedly occur less frequently than formerly";[5] and, two years later, another Washington psychiatrist, Henry Laughlin, was still more emphatic, asserting that "such symptoms are rarely seen in the civilian practice of psychiatry."[6] Scarcely a decade on, Ilza Veith, who interpreted the entire history of the disease through a psychoanalytic lens, complained, as she drew her discussion to a close, about "the nearly total disappearance of the illness." It had become, she thought, "an apparently infrequent disease"—ironically enough, according to her account, precisely because Freud had understood its dynamics so well, and had communicated his message so well, that "hysteria had become subjectively unrewarding...the 'old-fashioned' somatic expressions have become suspect among the more sophisticated classes, and hence most physicians observe that obvious conversion symptoms are now rarely encountered and, if at all, only among the uneducated of the lower social strata."[7]

"Where has all the hysteria gone?" asked the female analyst Roberta Satow.[8] Gone to its grave, said Étienne Trillat, "and taken its secrets with it."[9] Satow's query would soon find its echo in another mystery: "Where have all the psychoanalysts gone?" In 1970, with only a handful of exceptions, all the major departments of psychiatry in North America were headed by a psychoanalytically trained psychiatrist. A decade and a half later, virtually none of them was. Instead, neuroscience ruled the roost. It was a sudden and spectacular fall from grace, a story that surely includes elements of profound political miscalculation (a misreading by the analysts of the significance of the move to the neo-Kraepelinian reclassification of mental diseases, and the impact of that cataclysmic cognitive shift on the legitimacy of psychoanalytic approaches); the growing sense that psychoanalysis just did not work (and, not infrequently, diagnosed real organic disorders as neurotic illnesses, to sometimes disastrous effect); and, perhaps most notably of all, the psychopharmacological revolution (both via its direct effects, and through the massive infusion of Big Pharma money it brought in its train). That revolution massively affected the practice of psychiatry at many different levels: clinically; cognitively; organizationally; even politically. By the mid-1980s, American psychoanalytic training institutes, having previously been rigorous about excluding all but MDs from training analyses, were welcoming lay analysts for the first time, as the enrolment of the medically trained all but vanished.

For better or worse, we now live in a psychopharmacological age. Prozac and Valium, Thorazine and Zoloft, and a host of other psychoactive substances, are daily ingested by millions, and have made fortunes for those creating and peddling them to an ever expanding market of eager (and sometimes not-so-eager) consumers. Since 1980, when the American Psychiatric Association promulgated the third edition of its *Diagnostic and Statistical Manual* (DSM III), American psychiatry has achieved worldwide hegemony, and in many ways pills have replaced talk as the dominant response to disturbances of emotion, cognition, and behavior. Pharmaceutical corporations have underwritten the revolution, and have rushed to create and exploit a burgeoning market for an ever broader array of drugs aimed at treating some of the hundreds of "diseases" psychiatrists claim to be able to identify. And patients and their families have learned to attribute their travails to biochemical disturbances, to faulty neurotransmitters, and to genetic defects, and to look to their doctors for the magic potions that will produce better living through chemistry.

The re-biologization of psychiatry has been accompanied by what Mark Micale has wittily called the "exorcism" of hysteria from psychiatry—a systematic effort to root out the last lingering residues of psychiatry's Freudian misadventure. The lack of concern among psychoanalysts about problems of descriptive psychopathology had led them to ignore the formation in 1974 of the American Psychiatric Association's Task Force on Nomenclature and Statistics, the group charged with updating psychiatry's *Diagnostic and Statistical Manual* to accord with a forthcoming revision of the International Classification of Diseases (ICD). Early protests from Howard Berk that "*DSM* gets rid of the castle of neurosis and replaces it with a diagnostic Levittown"[10] were met with soothing words and swift action to marginalize him. The one psychoanalyst appointed to the panel found his suggestions routinely scorned and ignored, and resigned in protest. His departure was only one of a multitude of political miscalculations on the analysts' part. Just months before the publication of the Task Force's report, it finally dawned on some of them that the proposed document amounted to "a wholesale expurgation of psychodynamics from the psychiatric knowledge base."[11]

There was a flurry of protest. Threats were made to mobilize the membership to reject the new manual. Elaborate negotiations ensued. The analysts were thoroughly outmaneuvered. Meekly, they agreed to a "compromise": the term "'neurosis,' whatever the word signified, was psychoanalysts' bread and butter," and comprised those disorders, including the now rarely seen hysteria, that were at the core of their enterprise; but, rather than being reinstalled into the body of the manual (a step that would have compromised the neo-Kraepelinians' goals), it was agreed that the words "neurotic disorder" would be added in parentheses after the newly named "diseases" that had previously formed part of the kingdom of the neuroses. So it came to pass that "the appellative 'neurosis' and the clinical, psychodynamic tradition for which it stood had been marginalized to the relative obscurity of parentheses." And soon not even that: a further revision some seven years later eliminated the parenthetical additions. Hysteria and indeed the whole array of "neurotic" disorders had been carved up and thrust out of sight. As Donald Klein, a leading psychopharmacologist and one of the authors of the revolution, later gloated: "The neurosis controversy was a minor capitulation to psychoanalytic nostalgia."[12]

It is tempting to trace the residual nooks and crannies where bits and pieces of the old hysteria hang out, hidden from sight in the new neo-Kraepelinian consensus. After all, the various versions of the *Diagnostic and Statistical Manual* resemble the Yellow Pages in more than just their propensity to grow ever more elephantine as time goes by. (David Healy has pointed out that the number of psychiatric "illnesses" one can suffer from grew from 180 in the third edition, to 292 in the revised third edition, and to over 450 by the time the fourth edition appeared.) As in the Yellow Pages, if one looks diligently enough through the manual, one can find whatever one desires: in this case, the tools to pathologize virtually any species of human behavior, and categories and concepts that one can use in all sorts of creative fashions. "Shell shock" begat "combat exhaustion," which begat the politically contrived diagnosis of "post-traumatic stress disorder," or PTSD. Surely cases of classic conversion hysteria lurk under the disguise of the new scientistic categories: as "dissociative disorder: conversion type"; or as "histrionic personality type"; perhaps as "psychogenic pain disorder"; or under the catch-all categories of "undifferentiated somatoform disorder" or "factitious illness behavior"? That would suggest that hysteria has vanished as a medical diagnosis because of a fundamental redefinition of the psychiatric landscape, one that its enthusiasts compare to the replacement of superstition by science, and its critics see as more closely analogous to the recreation of the extraordinary and baroque nosologies that were a feature of eighteenth-century medicine.

The Canadian medical historian Edward Shorter has suggested a different explanation for hysteria's strange evolution. There exist, he suggests, repertoires of psychosomatic illness that are characteristic of particular cultures and particular epochs in our history. Throughout history, he suggests, the phenomenon of hysterical conversion can be found: the "flight into illness" via the transformation of acute emotional anxiety into physical symptoms, motivated by the secondary gains the sick role can provide. A particular cultural and social setting and the reigning medical theories of the day provide a symptom pool from which the unconscious mind selects the kinds of somatization that then manifest themselves: swooning in the eighteenth century; paralyses, gait disturbances, seizures, and retreats into the role of permanent nervous invalid in the nineteenth century; eating disorders and chronic fatigue in the twentieth century. "By defining certain symptoms as illegitimate," he claims, "a culture strongly encourages patients not to develop them or to risk being thought 'undeserving' individuals with no real medical problems. Accordingly, there is great pressure on the unconscious mind to produce only legitimate symptoms."[13]

There is another possibility, however. Perhaps hysteria is not dead after all? Perhaps Charcot was right when he insisted that "L'hystérie a toujours existé, en tous lieux et en tous temps."[14] Perhaps the disease that even those who insist on its reality concede is the very instantiation of lability, a chameleon-like disorder that can mimic the symptoms of any other, and that seems to mold itself to the culture in which it appears, has just assumed a different guise? And one not so very different, it may be, from the disorders Charcot and Freud encountered and described.

Shorter has suggested that the *grands gestes* of Charcot's Paris have been replaced by a more anodyne and elusive set of symptoms, chronic fatigue notable among them. Chronic fatigue syndrome has an obvious overlap with the neurasthenia of the late nineteenth century, and is a disorder that is similarly subjective and hard to disprove. Its sufferers insist, like other hysterics, that theirs is a real physical disorder, and, if it lacks the drama presented by the seizures, the hemi-paralyses, and the erotic writhings and moans of Charcot's patients, it nonetheless presents with an impressive array of bodily symptoms: sore throats, memory loss, aching muscles and heads, insomnia, general lassitude. Fearful of being labeled classic hysterical malingerers, its victims have often opted for labels that seem more distinctively and solidly medical: Epstein-Barr virus; fibromyalgia; or myalgic encephalomyelitis (grim sounding and serious, except when rendered in the form of its unfortunate acronym, ME). It has scarcely helped. Mainstream medicine has evinced skepticism, and the public at large has gleefully dismissed the disorder as "yuppie flu."

Bitterly, the fatigued denounce their critics, the worst-placed rattling their wheelchairs in lieu of shaking their fists, accusing doctors of being "lamentably ignorant of the most basic facts of the disease." Proudly they re-dedicated themselves to "the long uphill battle against ignorance and inertia."[15] Pesticides, hormones, chemicals, bacteria, viruses: something must surely be responsible for their suffering, and, if modern medicine pronounces itself unable to oblige with a physical account of their troubles, and proposes to ship them off to the tender mercies of the psychiatric profession, then they must seek help elsewhere. Some have opted for self-help or have turned to holistic practitioners, who are happy to display more sympathy and faith in the physical reality of their disorder, and to link it, as the nineteenth-century proponents of American nervousness once did, to the perils of civilization, only this time in the guise of a poisoned modern environment. Others have sought online support groups, where they can share their experiences and sense of grievance. The verbally and sometimes (ironic as that would be) almost physically violent response of the ME patients to the suggestion that their symptoms are psychosomatic, or "all in their heads," is a clue to what may have happened to other, more dramatic cases of hysteria. Such patients desperately want a neurological diagnosis. That diagnosis will validate the reality of their disorder, and legitimize their suffering, but the neurologists who have grown to professional maturity in the post-Charcot world evince little or no interest in their troubles. Pausing only long enough, in the most plausible of cases, to subject them to batteries of tests and scans before pronouncing them physically normal, they suggest these troublesome patients go to see a psychiatrist. But that is the last thing these patients want.

The neurologists' dismissal is not new. Bernard Sachs spoke for many of his neurological colleagues early in the twentieth century when he dismissed the hysterical as peripheral to the neurological enterprise:

> While hysterical and neurasthenic patients, and others of the same order, are numerous enough, their ailments and sufferings are, after all, less important than the sufferings of those who are afflicted with various forms of organic spinal disease, say tabes, primary lateral sclerosis, and the like. Let us try to do more for these patients…and do not let us waste too much energy on what people are pleased to call psychotherapy.[16]

The reluctance of most neurologists to entangle themselves with such cases has, if anything, increased with time. The attention devoted to hysteria and related complaints in neurological textbooks was reduced almost to vanishing point after 1950: "non-organic problems featured only as something to rule out when looking for neurological disease."[17]

Hysterical patients still present themselves in neurological waiting rooms, only to be turned away by doctors who have no interest in seeing or treating them. In the process, an age-old disorder becomes almost literally invisible. Shunned by the doctors they seek to consult to validate their symptoms, and defined out of existence by a pharmacologically oriented psychiatry (even were they willing to swallow their pride and accept the psychological roots of their discomforts), hysterics find themselves modern medicine's untouchables.

And yet—as Sir Aubrey Lewis once sagely remarked, "a tough old word like hysteria dies very hard. It tends to outlive its obituarists."[18]

GLOSSARY

ABREACTION a psychoanalytical term, referring to efforts to get a patient to relieve a traumatic experience under controlled conditions in order to purge it of its emotional charge

ALIENIST a replacement for the earlier English term "mad-doctor," derived from the French *alieniste*, and referring primarily to those medical practitioners who treated the mentally ill in institutional settings; there was strong resistance in the English-speaking world to the alternative label of "psychiatrist," originally a German coinage, until the early years of the twentieth century

AMYOTROPHIC LATERAL SCLEROSIS a degenerative disorder affecting motor neurons in both the brain and the spinal cord, primarily found among those over 50 and universally fatal, usually in six years or less; it produces progressive weakness and atrophy, and eventually an inability to breathe because of muscular paralysis

APHASIA an impaired ability to comprehend or express language in its written or spoken form, often, but by no means always, the aftermath of a stroke

APOPLEXY a sudden loss of neurological function, without convulsions, the product of hemorrhage, or constriction or obstruction of blood vessels in the brain

ASEPTIC SURGERY one of the key developments in surgery in the late nineteenth century, the attempt to prevent access by infecting organisms to surgical wounds, thus greatly reducing surgical complications and mortality

BAQUET a device employed by Anton Mesmer to permit multiple patients (as many as twenty-four patients) to be mesmerized simultaneously, consisting of a tub filled with water that had been charged with the animal magnetism emanating from Mesmer himself, with a polished metal cover, and metal rods protruding at intervals; by grasping these rods, patients could readily be "magnetized"

CATALEPSY decreased responsiveness to the external environment and profound inactivity, often with limbs remaining where they are placed (so-called waxy flexibility); often a symptom of psychosis, it may also be produced by drug toxicity

CEREBRAL PALSY a generic term for a group of non-progressive motor disorders of varying degrees of severity, ranging from defects in fine motor control to spasticity affecting all limbs, generally associated with brain damage prenatally, at birth, or during infancy

CHOREA involuntary, spasmodic movements that are forcible, rapid, and jerky, and markedly affect normal patterns of movement

CUPPING a widely employed technique in traditional medicine, using a so-called cupping glass and a tool to puncture the skin to draw blood from the body; its localized action was thought to permit the removal of congestion at a particular site

DEGENERATION a doctrine that originated among French psychiatrists in the last third of the nineteenth century and quickly spread internationally, proferring a biological explanation for all manner of social pathology (crime, alcoholism, mental illness, and more), and postulating the inheritance of acquired characteristics—in essence, it was as though evolution ran in reverse, so that, over a few generations, the civilized became the savage became the sub-human

DIATHESIS having an unusual susceptibility to certain diseases

EMMENAGOGUES chemical compounds that induce menstruation or miscarriage

FIBROMYALGIA tenderness and pain in the muscles, often associated with fatigue, sleep disturbances, stiffness, and headaches, all of which may be complicated by depression; often used as an alternative label for chronic fatigue syndrome, its etiology remains controversial and unclear

FISTULA an opening or connection between two internal organs that are normally separate, or between an internal organ and the surface of the body, that typically fails to heal

GLOBUS HYSTERICUS the sensation, common among hysterics, of a ball lodging in the throat or esophagus, interfering with respiration and swallowing, generally thought to have a psychological origin

HEMIANESTHESIA loss of sensation over one half of the body

HYPOCHONDRIA (THE HYP) for eighteenth-century physicians and lay people, a physical illness located in the region of the hypochondrium or diaphragm, the region traditionally regarded as the seat of melancholy; only gradually did the term acquire its modern meaning: the neurotic conviction that one is ill or bound to become ill in the very near future

ISSUE an incision designed to allow the discharge of blood or pus, a therapeutic technique widely employed in Hippocratic medicine

LOCOMOTOR ATAXIA a condition characterized by the degeneration of the sensory neurons, producing stabbing pains in the trunk, an unsteady gait, incontinence, impotence, and eventually death; a form of tertiary syphilis

MEDULLA more correctly medulla oblongata: a portion of the brain stem that lies between the pons, and the spinal cord below, and that plays an important role in controlling autonomic functions, such as breathing and blood pressure

MULTIPLE SCLEROSIS a chronic, degenerative, and incurable, but often episodic, disease of the central nervous system, characterized by mild to severe impairments of the nerves and muscles, bladder dysfunction, or disturbances of the visual field, the product of a patchy destruction of the myelin that surrounds and insulates nerve fibres; its etiology is unknown, and treatments are at best palliative

MYALGIC ENCEPHALOMYELITIS (ME) a congeries of symptoms of indeterminate origin, sometimes claimed to result from immune system dysfunction, or to be a post-viral fatigue syndrome, and often used as an impressive-sounding alternative to chronic fatigue syndrome; prominent complaints may include fatigue, persistent headache and malaise, visual disturbances, sleep disturbances, muscle pain, nausea, and mood changes and also irritability, depression, anger; its clinical status is controversial

NEO-KRAEPELINIAN refers to the movement in modern psychiatry from the late 1970s onwards to create explicit, operationalizable, and reliable diagnostic criteria to divide mental illness into an increasingly larger array of subcategories ("reliable" is here used in a technical sense: it means an approach that will generate a high degree of convergence among clinicians diagnosing independently, something that does not necessarily mean that the label they are conferring corresponds to a valid distinction in nature); Emile Kraepelin was a late-nineteenth-century German psychiatrist who developed a nosology or way of dividing up serious mental disorders that came to dominate Western psychiatry for generations

NOSOLOGY the classification of diseases in some systematic fashion

OVARIOTOMY the surgical removal of the ovaries

PARKINSON'S DISEASE a degenerative disorder of the central nervous system characterized by tremor and impaired muscular coordination, peculiarities of gait and posture, slowed movement and weakness, and partial paralysis of the face, named for the British physician, James Parkinson (1755–1824); it is linked to decreased dopamine production in the brain, and may be associated with cognitive deterioration in advanced cases

PARTURITION childbirth

PONS a knob-like protuberance at the front of the brain stem that lies between the medulla oblongata and the mid-brain; it relays sensory information, regulates respiration, and controls arousal

PSYCHOPHYSICAL PARALLELISM a doctrine, particularly associated with the nineteenth-century British neurologist John Hughlings Jackson, which holds that mental and bodily events occur in parallel series, but without causal interaction; mind and brain are allegedly precisely synchronized and correlated, even though independent of each other

SETONS threads, horsehair, or linen introduced beneath the skin and designed to provoke inflammation and the drainage of pus, widely used in traditional medicine to provide a pathway for noxious substances out of the body

TOURETTE'S SYNDROME a neurological disorder first described by Charcot's pupil and disciple Gilles de la Tourette in 1885; it is characterized by recurrent involuntary movements and neck jerks, often associated with vocal tics that may include grunts and barks, but especially streams of obscenities

NOTES

Prologue

1. Stephan Bradwell, "Mary Glover's Late Woeful Case, Together with her Joyfull Deliverance," Sloane MS 831, British Library, repr. in Michael MacDonald, *Witchcraft and Hysteria in Elizabethan London* (London: Routledge, 1991), 3.

2. Bradwell, "Mary Glover's Late Woeful Case," 3.

3. Bradwell, "Mary Glover's Late Woeful Case," 4.

4. Bradwell, "Mary Glover's Late Woeful Case," 4.

5. Bradwell, "Mary Glover's Late Woeful Case," 5–6.

6. Bradwell, "Mary Glover's Late Woeful Case," 7.

7. Bradwell, "Mary Glover's Late Woeful Case," 19.

8. Bradwell, "Mary Glover's Late Woeful Case," 21.

9. Bradwell, "Mary Glover's Late Woeful Case," 21.

Chapter 1

1. Quoted in Barbara Sicherman, "The Uses of a Diagnosis: Doctors, Patients, and Neurasthenia," *Journal of the History of Medicine and Allied Sciences,* 32 (1977), 41.

2. Edward Shorter, "The Reinvention of Hysteria," *Times Literary Supplement,* June 17, 1994, p. 26.

3. Eliot Slater, "Diagnosis of 'Hysteria'," *British Medical Journal,* 1 (1965), 1395–9.

4. Philip Slavney, *Perspectives on "Hysteria"* (Baltimore: Johns Hopkins University Press, 1990), 1–2.

5. I. S. Cooper, *The Victim is Always the Same* (New York: Harper and Row, 1976).

6. Charles Rosenberg, "The Therapeutic Revolution," in Charles Rosenberg and Morris Vogel (eds.), *The Therapeutic Revolution* (Philadelphia: University of Pennsylvania Press, 1979), 7.

7. George Rousseau, "A Strange Pathology: Hysteria in the Early Modern World," in Sander Gilman et al., *Hysteria beyond Freud* (Berkeley and Los Angeles: University of California Press, 1993), 107.

8. L. Targa (ed.), *Celsus on Medicine*, i (London: Cox, 1831), quoted in Ilza Veith, *Hysteria: The History of a Disease* (Chicago: University of Chicago Press, 1965), 21.

9. Edward Jorden, *A Briefe Discourse of a Disease Called the Suffocation of the Mother* (London: Windet, 1603), fo. 5^r, repr. in Michael MacDonald, *Witchcraft and Hysteria in Elizabethan London* (London: Routledge, 1991). (Foliation in this text is only on the front of each page, with the reverse left unpaginated. By convention, references to the front page are followed by an "r" for recto, and on the back by a "v" for verso.)

10. Jorden, *A Briefe Discourse*, fo. 1^v.

11. Jorden, *A Briefe Discourse*, fo. 2^r.

12. Jorden, *A Briefe Discourse*, fo. 2^r.

13. Stephan Bradwell, "Mary Glover's Late Woeful Case," in MacDonald, *Witchcraft*, 28.

14. Bradwell, "Mary Glover's Late Woeful Case," 29.

15. Jorden, *A Briefe Discourse*, title page.

16. Jorden, *A Briefe Discourse*, The Epistle Dedicatorie [the dedication], non-paginated.

17. Jorden, *A Briefe Discourse*, The Epistle Dedicatorie [the dedication], non-paginated.

Chapter 2

1. *Diary and Letters of Madam D'Arbly*, ed. C. F. Barrett (London: Coburn, Hurst and Blackett, 1854), iv. 239.

2. Thomas Willis, *Cerebri anatome* (London, 1764), 124.

3. Thomas Willis, *An Essay on the Pathology of the Brain and Nervous Stock* (London: Dring, Harper and Leigh, 1681), 76–8.

4. Willis, *An Essay on the Pathology*, 76–8.

5. William Harvey, *Exercitationes de generatione animalium* (London: Gardianis, 1651).

6. Willis, *An Essay on the Pathology*, 78.

7. Giovanni Battista Morgagni, *The Seats and Causes of Diseases Investigated by Anatomy*, ii (London: Millar, Cadell, Johnson and Payne, 1769), 628–9.

8. *The Entire Works of Dr Thomas Sydenham, Newly Made English*, ed. John Swan (London: Cave, 1742), 367–71.

9. *The Entire Works of Dr Thomas Sydenham*, ed. Swan, 374–5.

10. Nicholas Robinson, *A New System of the Spleen* (London: Bettesworth, Innys, and Rivington, 1729), 50.

11. Thomas Willis, *Two Discources Concerning the Soul of Brutes* (London: Dring, Harper, and Leigh, 1683), 206.

12. Willis, *Two Discources*, 206.

13. John Purcell, *A Treatise of Vapours, or, Hysterick Fits* (London, 1702), quoted in Richard Hunter and Ida McAlpine (eds.), *Three Hundred Years of Psychiatry* (Oxford: Oxford University Press, 1963), 289–91.

14. Bernard Mandeville, *A Treatise of the Hypochondriack and Hysterick Passions* (London: Leach, 1711).

15. Robinson, *New System*, 344–5.

16. Robinson, *New System*, 181–3.

17. Robinson, *New System*, 407–8.

18. Richard Blackmore, *A Treatise of the Spleen and Vapours: Or, Hypochondriacal and Hysterical Affections* (London: Pemberton, 1726), 96.

19. Blackmore, *A Treatise of the Spleen and Vapours*, 97.

20. Robinson, *New System*, 102.

Chapter 3

1. George Cheyne, *The English Malady* (London: Strahan and Leake, 1733), 343.

2. Cheyne's treatment of Catherine Walpole is the subject of a series of letters to Hans Sloane between 1720 and 1723, British Library, Sloane MS 4034, from which this and the following quotations are taken.

3. Richard Blackmore, *A Treatise of the Spleen and Vapours: Or, Hypochondriacal and Hysterical Affections* (London: Pemberton, 1726), pp. v–vi.

4. Cheyne, *The English Malady*, p. ii.

5. Cheyne, *The English Malady*, 52.

6. Cheyne, *The English Malady*, 182.

7. Cheyne, *The English Malady*, 174.

8. Cheyne, *The English Malady*, 49–50.

9. Cheyne, *The English Malady*, pp. i–ii.

10. Cheyne, *The English Malady*, 158–9.

11. Cheyne, *The English Malady*, 2–3.

12. Cheyne, *The English Malady*, 3.

13. Cheyne, *The English Malady*, 260.

14. Cheyne, *The English Malady*, 261.

15. Cheyne, *The English Malady*, 1.

16. James Boswell, *Boswell's Column* (London: Kimber, 1951), 42–3.

17. *The Letters of Samuel Johnson*, ed. R. Chapman (Oxford: Clarendon Press, 1974), ii. 245.

18. Jonathan Swift, "The Seventh Epistle of the First Book of Horace Imitated."

19. Alexander Pope, "Epistle to Arbuthnot."

20. Quoted in G. S. Rousseau, "A Strange Pathology," in Sander Gilman et al., *Hysteria beyond Freud* (Berkeley and Los Angeles: University of Calfornia Press, 1993), 167.

21. William Heberden, *Commentaries on the History and Cure of Diseases* (London: Payne, 1802), 227.

22. Cheyne, *The English Malady*, 79–80.

23. Roy Porter, *Mind Forg'd Manacles* (London: Athlone, 1987), 178.

24. William Heberden, *Medical Commentaries* (London: Payne, 1802), 233.

25. Quoted in Richard Hunter and Ida Macalpine (eds.), *Three Hundred Years of Psychiatry* (Oxford: Oxford University Press, 1963), 475.

26. Thomas Trotter, *A View of the Nervous Temperament* (London: Longman, 1807), 1.

27. Cheyne, *The English Malady*, 101.

28. Cheyne, *The English Malady*, 102.

29. Cheyne to Richardson, June 22, 1738, in *The Letters of Dr George Cheyne to Samuel Richardson*, ed. C. F. Mullett (Columbia, MO: University of Missouri Press, 1943), 38.

Chapter 4

1. David Rothman, *The Discovery of the Asylum* (Boston: Little, Brown, 1971).

2. Benjamin Rush, *Medical Inquires and Observations upon the Diseases of the Mind* (5th edn., Philadelphia: Grigg and Eliot, 1835), 103.

3. Richard Reece, *The Medical Guide* (London: Longman, 1802), 35.

4. W. Tyler Smith, "The Climacteric Disease in Women," *London Journal of Medicine*, 1 (1848), 607.

5. Robert Brudenell Carter, *On the Pathology and Treatment of Hysteria* (London: Churchill, 1853).

6. Brudenell Carter, *On the Pathology and Treatment*, 20.

7. Brudenell Carter, *On the Pathology and Treatment*, 33–4.

8. Brudenell Carter, *On the Pathology and Treatment*, 34.

9. Brudenell Carter, *On the Pathology and Treatment*, 46.

10. Brudenell Carter, *On the Pathology and Treatment*, 97.

11. Brudenell Carter, *On the Pathology and Treatment*, 55.

12. Brudenell Carter, *On the Pathology and Treatment*, 69.

13. Brudenell Carter, *On the Pathology and Treatment*, 108.

14. Brudenell Carter, *On the Pathology and Treatment*, 111.

15. Brudenell Carter, *On the Pathology and Treatment*, 114.

16. Brudenell Carter, *On the Pathology and Treatment*, 123.

17. Brudenell Carter, *On the Pathology and Treatment*, 151.

18. Carroll Smith-Rosenberg and Charles Rosenberg, "The Female Animal," *Journal of American History*, 60 (1973), 334.

19. George Man Burrows, *Commentaries on Insanity* (London: Underwood, 1828).

20. Horatio Storer, *Reflex Insanity in Women* (Boston: Lee and Shepard, 1871), 78.

21. Ornella Moscucci, *The Science of Woman* (Cambridge: Cambridge University Press, 1993), 104–5.

22. Storer, *Reflex Insanity*, 78–9.

23. Storer, *Reflex Insanity*, 80.

24. Dr Kellogg, quoted in Storer, *Reflex Insanity*, 86.

25. "Obituary: Mr Isaac Baker Brown, FRCS," *Lancet*, 1 (Feb. 8, 1873), 223.

26. "Obituary: Mr Isaac Baker Brown, FRCS," 223.

27. Isaac Baker Brown, *On the Curability of Certain Forms of Insanity … and Hysteria in Females* (London: Harwike, 1866), p. vi.

28. Baker Brown, *On the Curability of Certain Forms of Insanity*, 10.

29. Baker Brown, *On the Curability of Certain Forms of Insanity*, pp. 10, vi.

30. Baker Brown, *On the Curability of Certain Forms of Insanity*, 7–9.

31. Baker Brown, *On the Curability of Certain Forms of Insanity*, 17.

32. Baker Brown, *On the Curability of Certain Forms of Insanity*, 16.

33. Baker Brown, *On the Curability of Certain Forms of Insanity*, 70.

34. Elaine Showalter, *The Female Malady* (New York: Pantheon, 1985), 66.

35. "The Debate at the Obstetric Society," *British Medical Journal*, Apr. 6, 1867, pp. 407–8.

36. "The Week," *British Medical Journal*, Jan. 20, 1866, p. 77.

37. "Medical News: Spiritual Advice," *British Medical Journal*, Feb. 2, 1867, p. 119.

38. "Surgery for Lunatics," *British Medical Journal*, Feb. 9, 1867, p. 478.

39. Michael Clark, "The Rejection of Psychological Approaches to Mental Disorder in Late Nineteenth Century British Psychiatry," in A. Scull (ed.), *Madhouses, Mad-Doctors, and Madmen* (London: Athlone, 1981), 293.

40. "The Debate at the Obstetrical Society," *British Medical Journal*, Apr. 6, 1867, p. 388.

41. "The Debate at the Obstetrical Society," 409.

42. "The Debate at the Obstetrical Society," 396.

43. "The Debate at the Obstetrical Society," 407.

Chapter 5

1. E. C. Spitzka, "Reform in the Scientific Study of Psychiatry," *Journal of Nervous and Mental Diseases*, 5 (1878), 206–10.

2. Robert Battey, "Normal Ovariotomy," *Atlanta Medical and Surgical Journal*, 11 (1873), 1.

3. Quoted in Andrew Wynter, *The Borderlands of Insanity* (2nd edn., London: Renshaw, 1877).

4. William Goodell, "Clinical Notes on the Extirpation of the Ovaries for Insanity," *Transactions of the Medical Society of Pennsylvania*, 13 (1881), 640.

5. William Goodell, *Lessons in Gynecology* (Philadelphia: Davis, 1890), 395.

6. Wharton Sinkler, "The Remote Results of the Removal of the Tubes and Ovaries," *University Medical Magazine*, 4 (1891), 173.

7. D. Maclean, "Sexual Mutilation," *California Medical Journal*, 5 (1894), 38.

8. A. M. Hamilton, "The Abuse of Oophorectomy in Diseases of the Nervous System," *New York Medical Journal*, 57 (1893), 181; R. T. Edes, "Points in the Diagnosis and Treatment of Some Obscure Neuroses," *Journal of the American Medical Association*, 27 (1896), 1080.

9. Archibald Church, "Removal of the Ovaries and Tubes in the Insane and Neurotic," *American Journal of Obstetrics*, 28 (1893), 495; R. T. Edes, "The Relations of Pelvic and Nervous Diseases," *Journal of the American Medical Association*, 31 (1898), 1135.

10. Howard A. Kelly, "Conservatism in Ovariotomy," *Journal of the American Medical Association*, 26 (1896), 251.

11. Silas Weir Mitchell, *Rest in Nervous Disease: Its Use and Abuse* (A Series of American Clinical Lectures, ed. E. G. Seguin, vol. 1, no. 4; New York: Putnam, 1875), 94.

12. George Beard, *American Nervousness* (New York: Putnam, 1881), 17.

13. F. C. Skey, *Hysteria* (2nd edn., London: Longmans, 1867), 60.

14. Henry Maudsley, *The Pathology of Mind* (London: Macmillan, 1895), 37.

15. Beard, *American Nervousness*, 69.

16. Beard, *American Nervousness*, 70–1.

17. Beard, *American Nervousness*, 13.

18. Beard, *American Nervousness*, 26.

19. Janet Oppenheim, *Shattered Nerves: Doctors, Patients, and Depression in Victorian England* (Oxford: Oxford University Press, 1991), 141.

20. Silas Weir Mitchell, *Wear and Tear, or Hints for the Overworked* (5th edn., Philadelphia: Lippincott, 1891), 56.

21. Mitchell, *Wear and Tear*, 32.

22. Mitchell, *Wear and Tear*, 32.

23. Henry Maudsley, "Sex in Mind and Education," *Fortnightly Review*, 15 (1874), 466, 467.

24. Maudsley, "Sex in Mind and Education," 477.

25. Maudsley, "Sex in Mind and Education," 468, 479.

26. Maudsley, "Sex in Mind and Education," 76.

27. Silas Weir Mitchell, *Fat and Blood: An Essay on the Treatment of Certain Forms of Neurasthenia and Hysteria* (Philadelphia: Lippincott, 1899), 66.

28. Mitchell, *Fat and Blood*, 51.

29. Mitchell, *Fat and Blood*, 62–3.

30. Sir William Gull, "Anorexia Nervosa (Apepsia Hysterica, Anorexia Hysterica)," *Transactions of the Clinical Society of London*, 7 (1874), 22–8.

Chapter 6

1. J. M. Charcot, *Lectures on the Diseases of the Nervous System*, iii (London: New Sydenham Society, 1889), 3.

2. Quoted in Jan Goldstein, *Console and Classify* (2nd edn., Chicago: University of Chicago Press, 2001), 324.

3. Jules Falret, *Études cliniques sur les maladies mentales et nerveuses* (Paris: Ballière, 1890), 502.

4. Charcot, *Lectures*, iii. 14.

5. J. M. Charcot, *Leçons du mardi* (Paris: Bureaux du Progrès Médical, 1887), 481–2.

6. James Braid, *Neurypnology* (London: Churchill, 1843), 86.

7. Michael Clark, "The Rejection of Psychological Approaches to Mental Disorder in Late Nineteenth Century British Psychiatry," in A. Scull (ed.), *Madhouses, Mad-Doctors and Madmen* (London: Athlone, 1981), 290.

8. Ruth Harris, "Introduction" to the reprint edition of J. M. Charcot, *Clinical Lectures on Diseases of the Nervous System* (London: Routledge, 1991), p. xiv.

9. Charcot, *Lectures*, iii. 405.

10. Charcot, *Lectures*, iii. 13.

11. J. M. Charcot, "Leçon d'ouverture," *Progrès medical*, May 6, 1882, p. 336.

12. Charcot, *Lectures*, iii. 13.

13. Charcot, *Lectures*, iii. 18.

14. Quoted in Georges Didi-Huberman, *Invention of Hysteria* (Cambridge, MA: MIT Press, 2003), 87.

15. Axel Munthe, *The Story of San Michele* (London: Murray, 1930), 296, 302–3.

16. Quoted in Elaine Showalter, "Hysteria, Feminism and Gender," in Sander Gilman et al., *Hysteria beyond Freud* (Berkeley and Los Angeles: University of Calfornia Press, 1993), 311.

17. Quoted in Showalter, "Hysteria, Feminism and Gender," 311.

18. Thomas Laycock, *A Treatise on the Nervous Diseases of Women* (London: Longman, 1840).

19. J. M. Charcot, *Œuvres completes*, iii (Paris: Progrès Médical, 1890), 256.

20. J. M. Charcot, quoted in Elaine Showalter, *Hystories* (New York: Columbia University Press, 1997), 67.

21. Léon Daudet, *Memoirs*, quoted in Henri Ellenberger, *The Discovery of the Unconscious* (New York: Basic Books, 1970), 92.

22. Edmond de Goncourt, *Diary*, quoted in Ellenberger, *The Discovery of the Unconscious*, 92.

23. J. J. Déjerine, *Sémiologie des affections du système nerveux*, i (Paris: Masson, 1914), 561.

24. Munthe, *Story*, 302–3.

Chapter 7

1. George Makari, *Revolution in Mind* (London: Duckworth, 2008), 413, 474 (the latter a quote from Freud). This paragraph borrows its structure from the opening lines of Makari's excellent book.

2. *The Letters of Sigmund Freud*, selected and ed. Ernst Freud (New York: Basic Books, 1960), 184–5.

3. Josef Breuer and Sigmund Freud, *Studies on Hysteria*, trans. and ed. James Strachey (New York: Basic Books, 1957), 255, emphasis in the original.

4. Breuer and Freud, *Studies on Hysteria*, 160.

5. Breuer and Freud, *Studies on Hysteria*, 7, emphasis in the original.

6. Breuer and Freud, *Studies on Hysteria*, 294.

7. Breuer and Freud, *Studies on Hysteria*, 95.

8. Breuer and Freud, *Studies on Hysteria*, 185.

9. Quoted in Frank Sulloway, *Freud, Biologist of the Mind* (New York: Basic Books, 1979), 118.

10. Breuer and Freud, *Studies on Hysteria*, 17, emphasis in the original.

11. Josef Breuer and Sigmund Freud, *Studies on Hysteria*, in *Standard Edition of the Complete Psychological Works of Sigmund Freud*, trans. and ed. James Strachey, ii (reprint edn., London: Hogarth Press, 1981), preface, p. xxx.

12. Sigmund Freud, *An Autobiographical Study* (New York: Norton, 1963), 15–16.

13. Sigmund Freud, *Five Lectures on Psycho-Analysis* (New York: Norton, 1989), 6–7.

14. Freud, *Five Lectures*, 58.

15. Freud to Fliess, repr. in *The Origins of Psychoanalysis: Letters, Drafts and Notes to Wilhelm Fliess, 1887–1902*, ed. Marie Bonaparte, Anna Freud, and Ernst Kris (Garden City, NY: Doubleday, 1957), 76.

16. Quoted in Jeffrey Masson, *The Assault on Truth* (New York: Penguin, 1985), 9.

17. Sigmund Freud, "Fragment of a Case of Hysteria," in *Standard Edition of the Complete Psychological Works of Sigmund Freud*, trans. James Strachey, vii (reprint edn., London: Hogarth Press, 1981), 113.

18. Freud, "Fragment of a Case of Hysteria," 34.

19. Erik Erikson, quoted in Patrick Mahony, *Freud's Dora: A Psychoanalytic, Historical, and Textual Study* (New Haven: Yale University Press, 1996), 148–9.

Chapter 8

1. Max Weber to Marianne Weber, quoted in Hans Gerth and C. Wright Mills (eds.), *From Max Weber* (London: Routledge, 1991), 22.

2. Quoted in Barbara Tuchman, *The Guns of August* (New York: Random House, 2004), 141.

3. Quoted in Ben Shephard, *A War of Nerves* (Cambridge, MA: Harvard University Press, 2001), 18.

4. Quoted in John Keegan, *The First World War* (London: Pimlico, 1999), 390.

5. John T. MacCurdy, "War Neuroses," *Cornell University Medical Bulletin*, 7 (1918), 21.

6. Charles Mercier, *A Textbook of Insanity and Other Mental Diseases* (2nd edn., London: Allen and Unwin, 1914), 17

7. Quoted in Marc Roudebush, "A Battle of Nerves," in Mark Micale and Paul Lerner (eds.), *Traumatic Pasts* (Cambridge: Cambridge University Press, 2001), 261.

8. Paul Lerner, "From Traumatic Neurosis to Male Hysteria," in Micale and Lerner (eds.), *Traumatic Pasts*, 150–6.

9. Quoted in Lerner, "From Traumatic Neurosis to Male Hysteria," 156.

10. Lerner, "From Traumatic Neurosis to Male Hysteria," 158, 162.

11. Janet Oppenheim, *Shattered Nerves: Doctors, Patients, and Depression in Victorian England* (Oxford: Oxford University Press, 1991), 309.

12. MacCurdy, "War Neuroses," 6.

13. Quoted in Shephard, *War of Nerves*, 87–8.

14. Harvey Cushing, *From a Surgeon's Journal, 1915–1918* (Boston: Little, Brown, 1936), 489.

15. Quoted in Linda McGreey, *Bitter Witness: Otto Dix and the Great War* (New York: Lang, 2001), 304.

16. Shephard, *War of Nerves*, 63.

17. Quoted in Daniel Hipp, *The Poetry of Shell Shock* (Jefferson, NC: McFarland, 2005), 31.

18. Thomas Salmon, *The Care and Treatment of Mental Diseases and War Neuroses* (New York: National Committee for Mental Hygiene, 1917), 25.

19. Paul Lerner, *Hysterical Men* (Ithaca, NY: Cornell University Press, 2003), 102.

20. Roudebush, "A Battle of Nerves," 262.

21. Quoted in Roudebush, "A Battle of Nerves," 269.

22. Quoted in Elaine Showalter, *The Female Malady* (New York: Pantheon, 1985), 176–7.

Chapter 9

1. Étienne Trillat, *Histoire de l'hystérie* (Paris: Seghers, 1986), 274.

2. Carroll Smith-Rosenberg, "The Hysterical Woman," in *Disorderly Conduct: Visions of Gender in Victorian America* (New York: Knopf, 1985), 17.

3. Ellen Herman, *The Romance of American Psychology* (Berkeley and Los Angeles: University of California Press, 1995), 89.

4. Albert J. Glass, "Lessons Learned," US Army Medical Department, *Neuropsychiatry in World War II* (Washington: Government Printing Office, 1966), ii. 999–1000.

5. Paul Chodoff, "A Re-Examination of Some Aspects of Conversion Hysteria," *Psychiatry*, 17 (1954), 76.

6. Henry Laughlin, *The Neuroses in Clinical Practice* (Philadelphia: Saunders, 1956).

7. Ilza Veith, *Hysteria: The History of a Disease* (Chicago: University of Chicago Press, 1965), 273–4.

8. Roberta Satow, "Where Has All the Hysteria Gone?" *Psychoanalytic Review*, 66 (1979), 463–77.

9. Trillat, *Histoire*, 274.

10. Quoted in Stuart Kirk and Herb Kutchins, *The Selling of DSM: The Rhetoric of Science in Psychiatry* (New York: Aldine de Gruyter, 1992), 108.

11. Mitchell Wilson, "DSM III and the Transformation of American Psychiatry: A History," *American Journal of Psychiatry*, 150 (1993), 407.

12. Quoted in Wilson, "DSM III and the Transformation of American Psychiatry," 407.

13. Edward Shorter, *From Paralysis to Fatigue* (New York: Free Press, 1992), p. x.

14. Quoted in Trillat, *Histoire*, 272.

15. Simon Weseley, "New Wine in Old Bottles: Neurasthenia and 'ME,'" *Psychological Medicine*, 20 (1990), 39.

16. Bernard Sachs, "Commentary on 'The Attitude of the Medical Profession toward the Psychotherapeutic Movement,' by E. W. Taylor," *Journal of Nervous and Mental Diseases*, 40 (1908), 405.

17. Jon Stone, Russell Hewett, Alan Carson, Charles Warlow, and Michael Sharpe, "The 'Disappearance' of Hysteria: Historical Mystery or Illusion," *Journal of the Royal Society of Medicine*, 101 (2008), 12–18.

18. Aubrey Lewis, "The Survival of Hysteria," *Psychological Medicine*, 5 (1975), 9–12.

FURTHER READING

Even as cases of hysteria have become rather thin on the ground, and the disorder has been abandoned by the medical profession, historians and literary scholars have developed a renewed fascination for the subject (rather as psychoanalysis has essentially become extinct as a part of mainstream, re-biologized psychiatry, but has clung to life among anthropologists and literary types, who continue to insist that Freud is not an intellectual corpse). This generation of hysteria scholars sometimes refer to themselves as "the new hysterians," and their work has been catalogued in exhaustive detail by Mark Micale. His historiographic labors, many of them gathered in *Approaching Hysteria* (Princeton: Princeton University Press, 1995), are an obvious starting place for someone seeking a guide to this body of work.

The first to attempt a global history of the disorder was Ilza Veith. Her *Hysteria: The History of a Disease* (Chicago: University of Chicago Press, 1965) now seems a charming relic of an earlier age. Written at the height of the psychoanalytic dominance of American psychiatry, it interprets history relentlessly through a Freudian lens, damning biological speculations about hysteria, and praising those wise enough to anticipate aspects of Freudian theory. Though it surveys a vast terrain, it does so unreliably, constantly viewing the past through an anachronistic lens. That its own theoretical stance has now lost favor only makes its biases and limitations stand out in clearer relief. Étienne Trillat has served as hysteria's francophone historian, and his *Histoire de l'hystérie* (Paris: Seghers, 1986) contains much that is valuable, despite its inadequate coverage of many developments outside the French context. More recently, Sander Gilman, Helen King, Roy Porter, George Rousseau, and Elaine Showalter's *Hysteria beyond Freud* (Berkeley and Los Angeles: University of California Press, 1993) has traversed a grand historical territory, from Ancient Greece to the present. Characteristically certain of himself, Edward Shorter has looked broadly at psychosomatic illness in the modern age in *From Paralysis to Fatigue* (New York: Free Press, 1992). In related fashion, Showalter's *Hystories* (New York: Columbia University Press, 1997) treats such modern phenomena as chronic fatigue syndrome, recovered memory, multiple personality syndrome, and so forth as examples of modern hysterical epidemics.

For much of its history, hysteria was a prisoner of gender. Historians belatedly awoke to the need to make this a topic of inquiry in the 1980s. Elaine Showalter's *The Female Malady* (New York: Pantheon, 1985) remains fresh and provocative. The significance of male hysteria, a topic to which she gives more than glancing attention, has since been further explored by such writers as Paul Lerner and Mark Micale, both of whose books, confusingly, go by the title *Hysterical Men* (Ithaca, NY: Cornell University Press, 2003; New Haven: Yale University Press, 2008), though one deals with Charcot and *fin de siècle* Paris, and the other with shell shock among German soldiers in the First World War. Ranging widely on more than just hysteria, Lisa Appignanesi's *Mad, Bad, and Sad: A History of Women and the Mind Doctors from 1800 to the Present* (London: Virago, 2008) is nonetheless well worth reading.

Michael Macdonald's *Witchcraft and Hysteria in Elizabethan London* (London: Routledge, 1991) contains reprints of some key texts and a masterful introduction setting them in their contemporary contexts. It can be usefully supplemented by D. P. Walker's *Unclean Spirits* (Philadelphia: University of Pennsylvania Press, 1981). Richard Hunter and Ida Macalpine were the first to suggest that George III suffered from porphyria, and their *George III and the Mad Business* (London: Allen Lane, 1969) remains the most comprehensive discussion of the king's illness. On Cheyne, both Roy Porter's "Introduction" to the facsimile edition of Cheyne's *The English Malady* published by Routledge in 1991, and Anna Guerini's *Obesity and Depression in the Enlightenment* (Norman, OK: University of Oklahoma Press, 2000), are very useful, as is Cheyne's published correspondence with the Countess of Huntingdon and with Samuel Richardson (*The Letters of George Cheyne to the Countess of Huntingdon*, ed. C. F. Mullett (San Marino, CA: Huntington Library, 1940); *The Letters of Dr George Cheyne to Samuel Richardson*, ed. C. F. Mullett (Columbia, MO: University of Missouri Press, 1943)). On the eighteenth-century context more generally, Roy Porter's *Mind Forg'd Manacles* (London: Athlone, 1987) provides a useful overview, as does George Rousseau's rather rambling essay in *Hysteria beyond Freud*. My own *The Most Solitary of Afflictions* (New Haven: Yale University Press, 1993) tries to place nervous disorders in the broader context of changing attitudes towards madness. For a discussion of Mesmer and his times, see Robert Darnton, *Mesmerism and the End of the Enlightenment* (Cambridge, MA: Harvard University Press, 1968); and, on Victorian mesmerism, see Alison Winter, *Mesmerized* (Chicago: University of Chicago Press, 2000).

For the Victorian age more generally, Janet Oppenheim's *Shattered Nerves: Doctors, Patients, and Depression in Victorian England* (Oxford, Oxford University Press, 1991) provides a nuanced and balanced view of male and female nervous complaints, neither absolving Victorian medics of their prejudices, nor painting them in universally dark colors. Charles Rosenberg has examined the career of George Beard and the emergence of neurasthenia in an essay reprinted in his *No Other Gods* (2nd edn., Baltimore: Johns Hopkins University Press, 1997). Jan Goldstein's *Console and Classify* (2nd edn., Chicago: University of Chicago Press, 2001) provides a useful overview of French psychiatry in the nineteenth century. Ruth Harris's lively introduction to a reprint edition of Charcot's *Clinical Lectures on the Nervous System* (London: Routledge, 1991) covers considerable ground in a short space, and can be usefully supplemented by Henri Ellenberger's essay in his *Beyond the Unconscious* (Princeton: Princeton University Press, 1993), by the relevant chapter in Trillat's *Histoire de l'hystérie*, and by Mark Micale's *Hysterical Men*. For the most comprehensive study in English of Charcot's career, see Christopher Goetz, Michel Bonduelle, and Toby Gelfand, *Charcot: Constructing Neurology* (Oxford: Oxford University Press, 1995).

For Freud, of course, the problem is not a shortage of secondary works, but an overwhelming flood that shows no signs of abating. Psychiatry may have moved on. The publishing industry has not. Particularly useful, in my view, is George Makari's *Revolution in Mind* (London: Duckworth, 2008), wide-ranging and not overly polemical. Breuer and Freud's *Studies on Hysteria*, trans. and ed. James Strachey (New York: Basic Books, 1957), is, of course, an ur-text. For largely sympathetic re-examinations of Freud's famous clinical cases, see Lisa Appignanesi and John Forrester, *Freud's Women* (London: Orion, 2005). Albrecht Hirschmüller, *The Life and Work of Josef Breuer: Physiology and Psychoanalysis* (New York: New York University Press, 1989) provides fresh research on the real history of Anna O.; and for a wide-ranging psychoanalytic re-examination of the case of "Dora," see Patrick Mahony, *Freud's Dora: Psychoanalytic, Historical, and Textual Study* (New Haven: Yale University Press, 1996).

The connections of hysteria and trauma are surveyed in a collection of essays edited by Mark Micale and Paul Lerner (eds.), *Traumatic Pasts* (Cambridge: Cambridge University Press, 2001). Some of these essays examine the psychiatric casualties of the First World War in cross-national context. The single best treatment of shell shock and military psychiatry is Ben Shephard's *A War of Nerves* (Cambridge, MA: Harvard University Press, 2001). It is worth reading Charles Myers's original essay on the subject, "A Contribution to the Study of Shell Shock," *Lancet*, 1 (1915), 316–20, as well as his later monograph, *Shell Shock in France, 1914–1918* (Cambridge: Cambridge University Press, 1940). Paul Lerner's *Hysterical Men* is useful for the German context, and Martin Stone's essay "Shell Shock and the Psychiatrists," in W. F. Bynum, R. Porter, and M. Shepherd (eds.), *The Anatomy of Madness*, ii (London: Tavistock, 1985), provides some insight into English developments. John Keegan's classic *The First World War* (London: Pimlico, 1999) gives the reader some sense of the hell that was trench warfare, and the blunderings (and worse) of the generals and politicians.

For later developments, a two-part essay of mine, to appear in *History of Psychiatry* in 2010, explores some aspects of the rise and decline of psychoanalysis in post-Second World War America. For a participant's perspective, see Joel Paris, *The Fall of an Icon: Psychoanalysis and Academic Psychiatry* (Toronto: University of Toronto Press, 2005). The critical events surrounding the creation of the third edition of the American Psychiatric Association's *Diagnostic and Statistical Manual* are examined in Stuart Kirk and Herb Kutchins, *The Selling of DSM: The Rhetoric of Science in Psychiatry* (New York: Aldine de Gruyter, 1992), and in Mitchell Wilson, "DSM III and the Transformation of American Psychiatry: A History," *American Journal of Psychiatry*, 150 (1993), 399–410. For the key insider's account of the out-witting of the psychoanalysts over the exclusion of "neurosis" from the DSM, see Ronald Bayer and Robert Spitzer, "Neurosis, Psychodynamics, and DSM III," *Archives of General Psychiatry*, 42 (1985), 187–95. David Healy's *The Anti-Depressant Era* (Cambridge, MA: Harvard University Press, 1998) is a sophisticated account of the impact of psychopharmacology on the conceptualization as well as the treatment of mental illness in the late twentieth century. Gail MacLean and Simon Wessely provide a sobering look at "Professional and Popular Views of Chronic Fatigue Syndrome," *British Medical Journal*, 308 (Mar. 19, 1994), 776–7, which provides telling evidence of just how controversial the interpretation of this disorder has become.

In writing this book, I have drawn, of course, on a much wider range of scholarship than is contained in this list. Some of those debts are acknowledged—inadequately—in the notes. Many others do not receive even that courtesy. For that, I have to blame the pressures of space, and the impossibility of acknowledging fully the extent of one's debts in a work of synthesis like this one. Like many another author, I am lucky the debtor's prison is a thing of the past, and I hope those I have silently drawn upon are in a forgiving mood. For kind assistance of a more informal sort, I would like to thank Stephen Cox, Mark Micale, Gerald Grob, and Allan Horwitz. Above all, my thanks to William and Helen Bynum, general editors of this series, for commissioning me to write a book I have had a lot of fun writing; and for their careful scrutiny of, and constructive comments on, various drafts. They have done their best to save me from errors, and I alone am responsible for the ones that remain.

INDEX